I AM NORMA KAMALI INVINCIBLE

NORMA KAMALI
I AM INVINCIBLE

WITH SARAH BROWN

ABRAMS, NEW YORK

I DEDICATE THIS BOOK TO MY MOTHER . . .

SHE SEEMED ECCENTRIC, AND TIRELESS, IN HER COMMITMENT TO CREATIVITY; SHE PRACTICED A HEALTHY LIFESTYLE IN WAYS NO ONE ELSE UNDERSTOOD, AND STELLA WAS SURE THAT ANYTHING WAS POSSIBLE.

I HAVE BECOME HER.

TABLE
OF CONTENTS

I AM INVINCIBLE

WHEN I FEEL **EMPOWERED** AND WHEN

I AM **HEALTHY** I AM **STRONG** AND THEN

I CAN **DO** ALL THE THINGS I **NEED** TO DO

TO **REACH** THE **GOALS** I NEED TO REACH

IN ORDER TO **FULFILL** MY BIG **DREAMS**

THAT ARE AS **BIG** AS THE **WORLD** AND AS

OPTIMISTIC AS MY MIND CAN **IMAGINE**

I WILL **AGE WITH POWER** AND INFLUENCE

CHANGE BECAUSE **I KNOW MY PURPOSE**

This is my personal mantra and has been for as long as I can remember.

This book started out as a gift to a friend on her fiftieth birthday. A group of women were having a party for her, and all the gifts were meant to address the fifty-year mark in some way. I gave her a small leather-bound Moleskine notebook with my "50 Tips on Turning 50!" I was amazed at the reaction. I received texts, emails, and follow-up calls from many of the guests, asking me to make my book available. So here we are! That original book evolved and now is written for all women at every stage of their lives. This is my gift to you. Sleep, diet, and exercise are my Three Pillars. This is the healthy lifestyle you will see referenced in these pages over and over again. Together, these pillars energize and restore body and mind.

Each decade in a woman's life teaches and informs her ability to reach her potential. This is achieved through building self-esteem, recognizing and celebrating the authentic self, and living with purpose. I believe embracing a healthy lifestyle—which may entail rethinking lifetime habits—is key to how you look and feel. I began my career more than fifty years ago, and I still ride life's ups and downs. I was married at nineteen and divorced by twenty-nine. With ninety-eight dollars to my name, I left my husband and the business we created together behind, but I kept my soul. I never believed myself to be a businessperson, but surprisingly, I feel comfortable in the role. I work out every day. I have been meditating since 1970. I met my soul mate when I was sixty-five. I use my Scrabble app as an escape, and if there is a dance party, I am there. I believe the more you do, the more you can do. Five decades of failures and successes give me mountains of experience to impart. The way I have learned to live my life is proving ever more important to me now, as I finish writing this book during a worrisome time of uncertainty and unprecedented change. I am leaning on the good habits I have made in order to stay healthy and fortify my immune system, and am finding creative ways to pivot in order to adapt my business, quickly solve problems, look for the bright side, rise to the challenges, meaningfully connect with people, and keep living my purpose.

In this book are the practices I have researched and developed over many years, aided by the wisdom and insight from respected experts and pioneering industry leaders I have been fortunate to meet. This is what works for me, and I hope it will be helpful to you, too. If you have questions about how to incorporate certain advice or methodologies into your own life, consult with a doctor, nutritionist, trainer, or other healthcare professional about designing a plan that works best for you.

I am grateful for all I have learned and for what I am able to pass along to you. I am honored to share the professional and personal transitions I have made, the research I have done, and my ideas about how to move through the decades and age with power!

—**NORMA KAMALI**

NORMALIFE

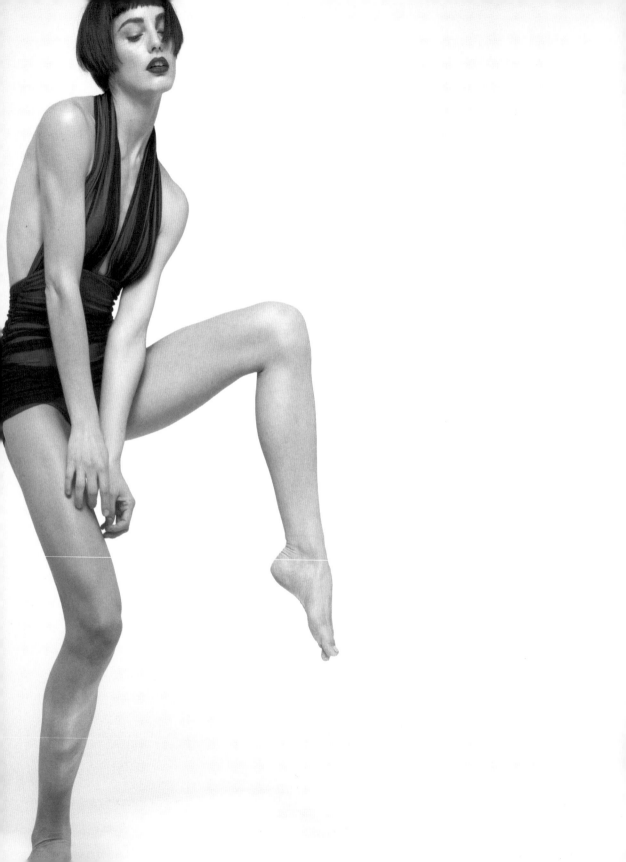

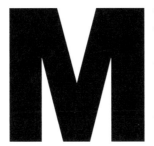**M**y thoughts about lifestyle are really simple: If you can control the quality of your life, why not do it? You can design your lifestyle to create the outcome you desire. NORMALIFE is my philosophy for living. It is built around the Three Pillars—sleep, diet, exercise—and the simple things everyone can do to maintain balance, happiness, and good health. For me, it is a state of mind. It is about making deliberate choices that become ingrained good habits, all of which make it easier to stay on track and to defuse difficult situations that otherwise might set one back. These are the things that work for me; I hope they will work for you, too.

A healthy lifestyle is an achievable concept. It may require some effort, some planning, and at times some willpower, but it doesn't have a price tag and it is not exclusive. Exercise is free. Singing, dancing, and laughing are free. Meditation is free, and so is sleep.

My early introduction to health and well-being was memorable and is still quite vivid.

When I was a kid, my mother (who lived from 1915 to 2002) would start juicing at six o'clock each morning. We lived in the smallest apartment in New York City, which she'd made even smaller by separating spaces so my brother and I had our own bedrooms. My space was two feet away from the vibrating steel juicer, which, by the way, was the size of a car engine and sounded as loud. She had supplements all over the house and herbs growing on every windowsill. From these shelves packed with greens, she'd snip mint leaves for tea and parsley for stomachaches, and incorporate all of them into our meals as flavorful ingredients. She gave us oil of oregano when we were sick and used olive oil for absolutely everything. This was the fifties, and my mother was what folks might have labeled "eccentric" at the time for practicing these alternative approaches to wellness. Literally no one else's mom was doing anything like this, and I would think to myself, *What is she doing?*

Now I am so grateful for her influence. Through my mother's approach to life, I learned the concept of timelessness: What works through the ages always works. I am very much aware of how timelessness is a dominant theme in everything I do, from the designs I create to the ingredients I source.

My commitment to learning more about a healthy lifestyle as an adult was motivated by the loss of my very dear friends to AIDS in the 1980s. How could I lose my two best friends in such a short period of time?

Gone!

The explanation for these countless deaths was that the immune system could no longer protect the body once it became compromised. I sought out information (no Google then; real research, old-school!), and in time I found pockets of knowledge in California, New Mexico, and Arizona. Work was being done rethinking the health and wellness status quo, and alternative practices for building a strong immune system were being developed. I changed how I was living and never looked back.

I've learned that the mind-body connection is a powerful source of well-being. We have the ability to create positive outcomes with an assortment of grounding practices. I find meditation and breathwork particularly effective for balance and stress release. When you use breath, you can manifest physical endurance and strength and—as in childbirth, for example—summon the ability to move beyond pain. Meditation is so helpful to me that in my fantasy it should be required for all Americans at a prescribed time daily. I was so pleased when my staff expressed an interest in meditation. Now, every day at twelve-thirty P.M., we close the company for a thirty-minute break. Some of my team sits yogi-style, some sit in a chair, some lie on mats, and sometimes there's snoring, and all of the above is okay.

Yoga, tai chi, and Gyrokinesis are great examples of active meditation that support the restorative process. Acupuncture helps open blockages throughout the body to increase the flow of energy. I love it for treating ailments, reducing stress, and invigorating my mind and body. Acupuncture's cumulative effects are even better, so weekly visits are great for overall

THROUGH MY MOTHER'S APPROACH TO LIFE, I LEARNED THE CONCEPT OF TIMELESSNESS: WHAT WORKS THROUGH THE AGES ALWAYS WORKS.

well-being—and, if you're getting an acupuncture facelift, as I do, a perky face, too.

I discovered the acupuncture facelift twelve years ago during a trip to China. I was having tea with a group of girlfriends and noticed that everyone at the table had bright eyes and a certain glow and tone to their skin. It prompted me to ask why they all looked so good. They said they had just had acupuncture facelifts! Excuse me! I was scheduled to leave the next day, so I immediately went on the hunt for the top expert in the United States.

I asked my wellness contacts, traditional doctors and people I knew in the Chinese community, for their recommendations. One name kept coming up: Dr. Jingduan Yang, one of the country's leading authorities on Chinese medicine and a doctor of Western medicine, too, with degrees in psychiatry and neurology.

I drove two-plus hours to Philadelphia (actually, I had to hire a car service, because New York City girls don't drive!), where Dr. Yang worked at Thomas Jefferson University Hospital, researching advanced uses of acupuncture. He escorted me into his office and asked why I wanted to see him. I immediately blurted out, "I want an acupuncture facelift." To which he promptly responded, "Well, you are not going to get one!" *Yowza*. I restrained my disappointment and asked why not.

He was actually offended that I had minimized acupuncture, an ancient methodology that had been handed down through four generations of practitioners in his family. He explained the Chinese medicine tradition and its philosophies and technique. Oh my, I was taken aback but enthralled by his commitment and his belief in the benefits both long- and short-term. I asked if he would educate me if I came for weekly treatments. He was very obliging and looked pleased that I had an interest, especially knowing it would entail four hours round-trip for me each visit. I pushed a bit more and asked if I could record our sessions, and he agreed. So, every Thursday at two P.M. I would head to Philadelphia.

By the third treatment, he surprised me with an acupuncture facelift. At first I was frightened by the thought of so many needles, but they are sooo thin, and by the time the last needle was in place, I was sound asleep. When Dr. Yang woke me an hour later, I was refreshed, relaxed, and uplifted. I felt like I'd slept for a month.

I remember this first experience so clearly because it wasn't until the next day at work in our open-plan office that someone (by the way, no one knew where I was going each Thursday) said, "You look really good today." I went to the bathroom to take a look, and damn, yeah, I did look good. There was a visible difference in my face, as if I'd had the best night's sleep of my life, or had just come back from a stress-free vacation. Even better, I felt really good. Since then, Dr. Yang and I have written a book together based on our meetings, *Facing East*, which includes a handbook of sorts on acupuncture.

NORMALIFE is about taking care of yourself and others. It embraces ideas that encourage kindness.

I love to laugh. Humor is healing, and I find it is the best way to dissolve conflict. To me, comedians are geniuses because intelligent humor digs deep into our belief systems, our habits, and quite frankly our core. Humor makes us think and helps us reevaluate and better understand our similarities rather than focus on our differences. I have found Brits to be especially funny. Humor is part of who they are. When I visit the U.K.—London and especially Manchester, where I am often for business—I laugh all the time. You can be sure that anyone you see has thought about a funny story to tell, and as a result, meetings start with a good laugh.

A healthy sense of self begins with love. Love and self-love are not to be taken for granted. The only way to truly experience love is to be able to give it. However, in order to give love to others, we need to learn how to love ourselves first. Positive self-esteem based on how we feel about our mind, body, and soul is needed for self-love. If we haven't done work in the self-love area, there is a chance we are not as discriminating as we need to be, especially in relationships.

The incredible side effect of self-love is that it radiates like a silent signal that people respond to positively. When we value ourselves, we draw love to us that is based upon respect and admiration. This love is safe and on a deeper level. You attract people you deserve and opportunities you deserve when you choose a lifestyle that results in the best version of you.

That said, walking away is one of the most important things I've learned in my life. There is a time to walk away from a relationship or a difficult situation. This is when your integrity and self-esteem are challenged. Walking away—not storming away, just politely walking away—signifies being in control and aware of your worth.

YOU ATTRACT PEOPLE YOU DESERVE AND OPPORTUNITIES YOU DESERVE WHEN YOU CHOOSE A LIFESTYLE THAT RESULTS IN THE BEST VERSION OF YOU.

Most people don't walk away. They'll succumb to reasonable compromise. Everyone wants a relationship or a job or a goal in life to work toward, and often we will endure the consequences of things going wrong to avoid what we perceive to be failure.

Walking away can be a negotiating tool and the way to get what you want. But you have to be comfortable giving up what you have for what you could gain. Sometimes *before* you have to walk away is precisely *when* you have to walk away.

I walked away from my marriage to save my soul. I've walked away from unhealthy business relationships and from potential partnerships that could have supported growth and scale for my company, but that I recognized would most likely have impacted the authenticity of the brand and my dream to live a creative life. Walking away begins with a belief system you have in your head about your own value.

Finally, kindness is doing something for others with no expectation in return. Make it part of your everyday behavior. Make someone else happy as often as you can. Open doors for strangers; give up your seat. Offer to help folks you know and don't know. There are friends and family who need some hand-holding and attention when issues arise in their lives. Be there. The elderly may need shopping done or help with technology. There are kids who need tutoring, and the community needs volunteers. There are so many ways to meet people through volunteering and simple thoughtfulness. You will engage with people with different points of view on life, and this will teach tolerance and to not fear what you do not know. The more you do, the more people around you will do the same. It is contagious.

These are the tools for creating a life of happiness, fulfillment, accomplishment, and purpose. NK

LITTLE GIRLS WITH DREAMS BECOME WOMEN WITH VISION.

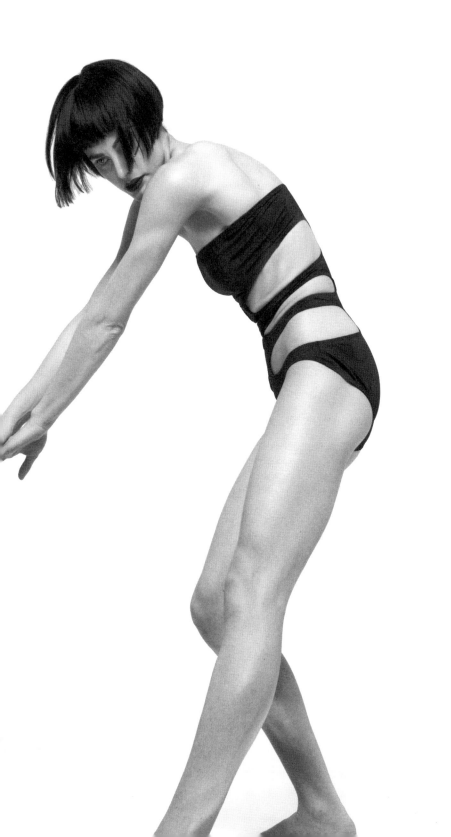

THE SPIRIT IS THE ESSENCE OF WHO WE ARE.

KEEPING IT STRONG AND OPEN IS AN IMPORTANT PART OF A LIFETIME. HOWEVER, THE SPIRIT SOMETIMES FADES EARLY, AND OUR LIFE PURPOSE IS CUT SHORT, UNFULFILLED. DO ALL YOU CAN TO KEEP IT ALIVE, EVEN UNDER EXTREME CHALLENGE.

KEEP YOUR SPIRIT ALIVE AND WELL.

SEE YOUR LIFE IN THE LONG DISTANCE.

IMAGINE WHAT'S AHEAD FOR YOU.

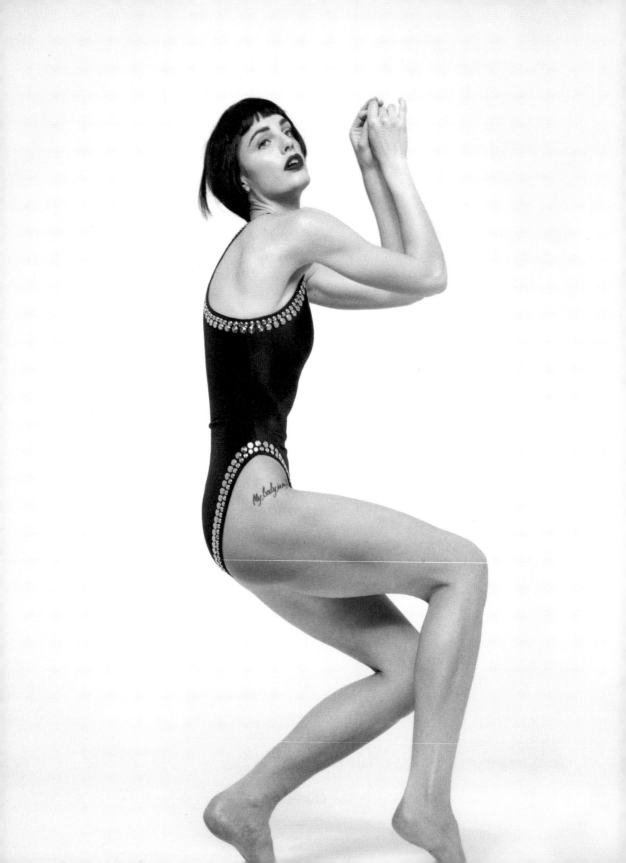

STAY INSPIRED.

BE CURIOUS.

LEARN SOMETHING NEW EVERY DAY.

ASK QUESTIONS.

OPEN YOUR MIND TO NEW IDEAS.

**THE RESULT IS
AN EVER-EVOLVING,
EXCITING YOU.**

CHANGE IS THE ESSENCE OF LIFE

BE WILLING TO SURRENDER WHO
YOU ARE FOR WHAT YOU CAN BECOME.
CHANGE IS VERY HARD FOR MANY PEOPLE,
BUT CHANGE IS INEVITABLE IN ALL OF OUR LIVES.
IT IS OFTENTIMES WHAT PROPELS US FORWARD.
IF YOU INITIATE CHANGE, YOU WILL HAVE
PROACTIVE MANAGEMENT OVER IT
AND THE OUTCOME IS MORE LIKELY TO BE POSITIVE.

HAVE SEX WITH YOUR PARTNER OR WITH YOURSELF

KEEP IN TOUCH.

LAUGH

SHARE + CREATE LAUGHTER EVERY DAY. FIND A COMEDY CHANNEL, MOVIE, OR VIDEO. SING AND DANCE.

FIND JOYOUS SITUATIONS OR MAKE THEM HAPPEN.

LAUGHING IS A GREAT WAY TO RELEASE STRESSFUL, NEGATIVE ENERGY . . . WE ALL FEEL GOOD AFTER A LAUGH, AND IT SPREADS JOY!

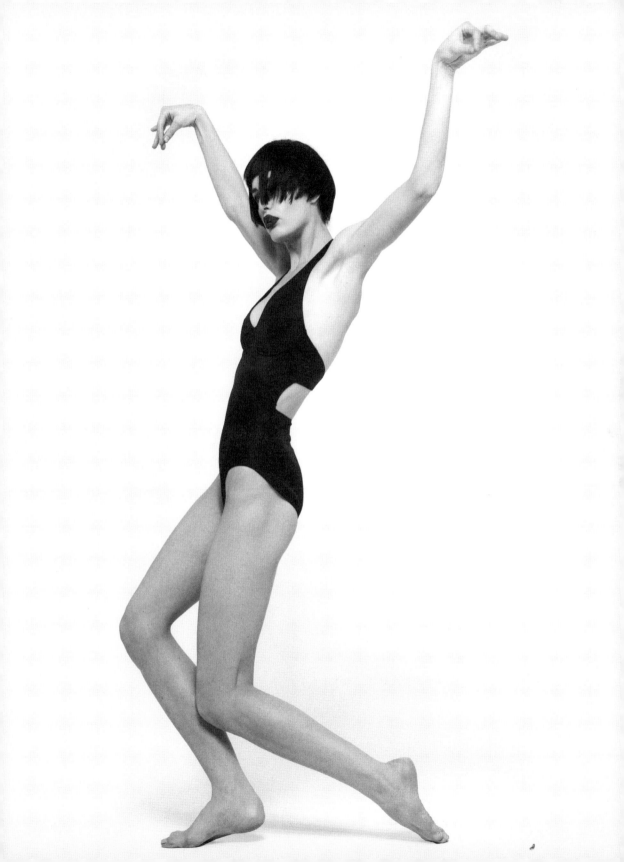

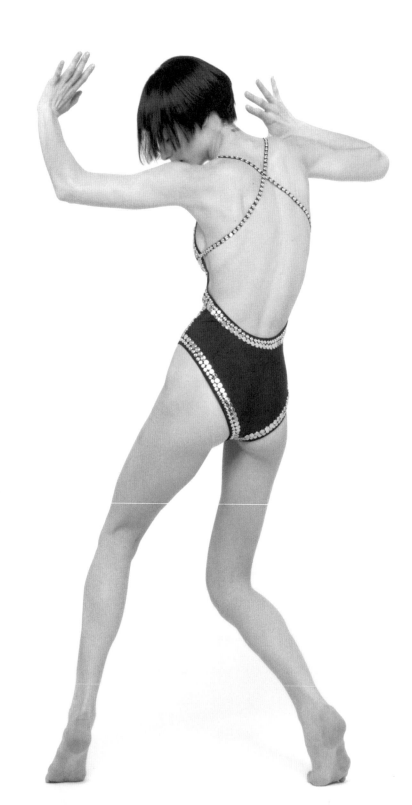

DANCING IS JOYOUS, AND IT IS FREE.

DANCING CREATES THE ULTIMATE RELEASE OF STRESS AND ENDORPHINS.

HOW YOU DANCE ONCE YOU LET YOURSELF GO IS AN EXPRESSION OF TOTAL FREEDOM.

KNOW YOUR HORMONE LEVELS.

THROUGHOUT PUBERTY, PREGNANCY, POST-PREGNANCY, PERIMENOPAUSE, AND MENOPAUSE, WOMEN RIDE A HORMONAL ROLLER COASTER. DIET AND EXERCISE ARE THE FIRST LINES OF DEFENSE FOR BALANCING HORMONES.

GET REGULAR HORMONAL CHECKUPS FROM YOUR DOCTOR OR WELLNESS PROVIDER TO BETTER ADDRESS THE EFFECT ON YOUR PHYSICAL AND MENTAL WELL-BEING.

OSTEOPOROSIS IS COMMON IN WOMEN, ESPECIALLY AS WE AGE. THE RISK OF DEVELOPING IT IS IMPACTED BY FACTORS LIKE BODY WEIGHT, ETHNICITY, DIET, AND FAMILY HISTORY.

WEIGHT-BEARING EXERCISES, GREEN VEGETABLES FOR NATURAL CALCIUM, AND CALCIUM SUPPLEMENTS THAT INCLUDE D_3, MAGNESIUM, VITAMIN C, AND SILICA FOR OPTIMAL ABSORPTION ARE ALL GOOD IDEAS.

BONE HEALTH IS IMPORTANT TO THINK ABOUT.

ASK YOUR DOCTOR TO CHECK YOUR CALCIUM ABSORPTION AND, AS YOU GET OLDER, YOUR BONE DENSITY, TOO.

AND HAVE A LOOK AT THE RECIPE FOR MY DAIRY-FREE BONE-HEALTH SMOOTHIE (P. 107), WHICH I DEVELOPED AS A WAY TO GET AS MUCH CALCIUM AS POSSIBLE THROUGH FOOD.

MASSAGE SUPPORTS
A STRONG IMMUNE SYSTEM
BY RELAXING AND
DESTRESSING THE BODY
AND MIND.

MASSAGES ARE MAGIC!

ACUPUNCTURE RELAXES; IT RELIEVES TENSION, MENSTRUAL CRAMPS, AND HOT FLASHES. IT CAN HELP PROMOTE FERTILITY AND SUPPORT YOUR IMMUNE SYSTEM FOR OVERALL WELL-BEING.

THINK ABOUT EASTERN MEDICINE AS AN OPPORTUNITY TO LOOK AT ANCIENT METHODS THAT WORK.

OUR SELF-WORTH
AND ACCOMPLISHMENTS
DEFINE WHO WE ARE.

ARE YOU WITH THE PERSON YOU DESERVE?

IT IS IMPORTANT FOR WOMEN TO
UNDERSTAND OUR VALUE SO THAT WE
ATTRACT AND ARE ATTRACTED TO THE
QUALITY OF PERSON WE DESERVE.

WHAT IS MOST IMPORTANT IN CHOOSING A MATE?

1 MAKES YOU LAUGH

2 HAS TONS OF MONEY

3 SHARES SAME
  POLITICAL PHILOSOPHY

4 IS VERY GOOD-LOOKING

5 THINKS YOU ARE THE BEST
  THING EVER

I ONCE DID AN INSTAGRAM SURVEY ON THE ABOVE. "THINKS YOU ARE THE BEST THING EVER" WON, WHILE "MAKES YOU LAUGH" CAME IN A CLOSE SECOND. THERE IS NO QUESTION THE TOP ANSWER IS THE MOST IMPORTANT.

BUT IN ORDER FOR YOU TO CONNECT TO A MATE WHO THINKS YOU ARE THE BEST THING EVER, AND TREATS YOU THAT WAY, YOU HAVE TO BELIEVE IT YOURSELF. THAT CAN TAKE SOME SERIOUS INTROSPECTION AND CONVERSATION WITH PEOPLE WHO LOVE YOU.

SUNBATHING IS NOT GOOD FOR YOU, ESPECIALLY WITHOUT SUNSCREEN.

BUT SUNSHINE IN MODERATION IS A GOOD SOURCE OF VITAMIN D, AN IMPORTANT VITAMIN FOR THE BODY. WHILE IT'S BEST FROM THE SUN, IT IS RECOMMENDED TO SUPPLEMENT VITAMIN D_3 IN THE WINTER OR WHEN YOU ARE NOT EXPOSED TO NATURAL SUNLIGHT. YOU CAN HAVE YOUR D_3 LEVELS MEASURED IN BLOOD TESTS, SO THE NEXT TIME YOU GO FOR A PHYSICAL, BE SURE TO ASK.

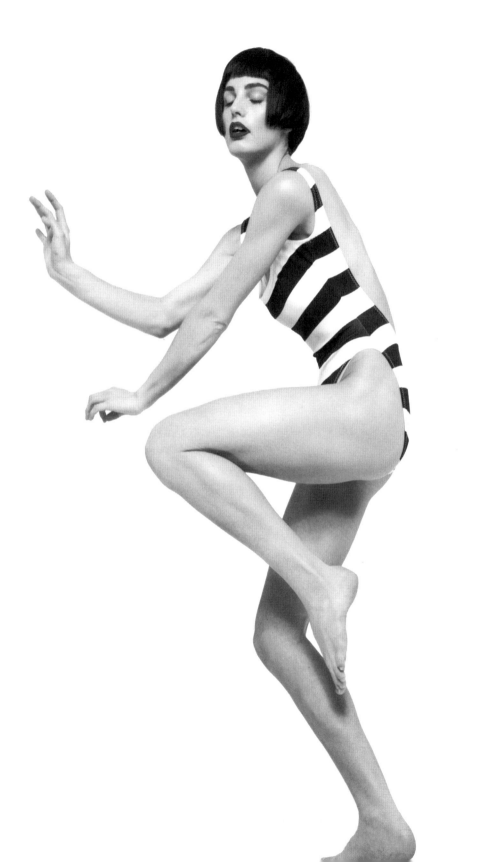

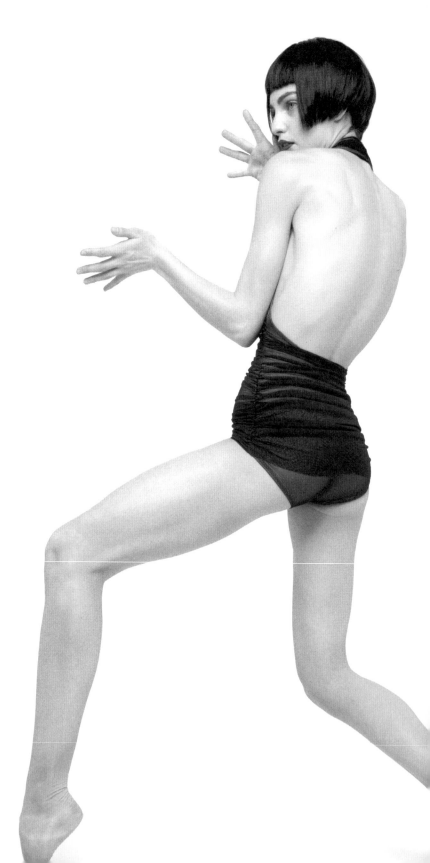

DON'T SMOKE.

A PERSON WHO SMOKES HAS TEN TIMES AS MANY WRINKLES AS A PERSON WHO DOES NOT. PLUS, IT'S REALLY BAD FOR YOU.

DUH.
DON'T SMOKE!

ZAP OUT TOXINS IN AN INFRARED SAUNA... A SUPER-IMMUNE BOOSTER.

THE IMMUNE SYSTEM WORKS MORE EFFICIENTLY WHEN TOXINS ARE REGULARLY RELEASED. ONE WAY TO RELEASE TOXINS IS VIA SWEAT.

I LOVE THE EXPERIENCE OF AN INFRARED SAUNA, WHICH HEATS THE BODY FROM WITHIN.

UNDERSTANDING DENTAL HEALTH IS IMPORTANT.

A FAMOUS SOCIALITE HAD HER TEETH CLEANED EVERY TWO WEEKS OF HER LIFE AND IN HER NINETIES HAD EVERY ORIGINAL TOOTH IN HER MOUTH. SHE WAS HEALTHY TO HER LAST DAY.

SCIENTISTS HAVE FOUND LINKS BETWEEN PERIODONTAL DISEASE AND HEART DISEASE, DIABETES, DEMENTIA, AND RHEUMATOID ARTHRITIS. THE BELIEF IS THAT ORAL BACTERIA CAN ENTER THE BLOODSTREAM AND INJURE MAJOR ORGANS.

VISIT THE DENTIST REGULARLY FOR PROFESSIONAL CLEANINGS.

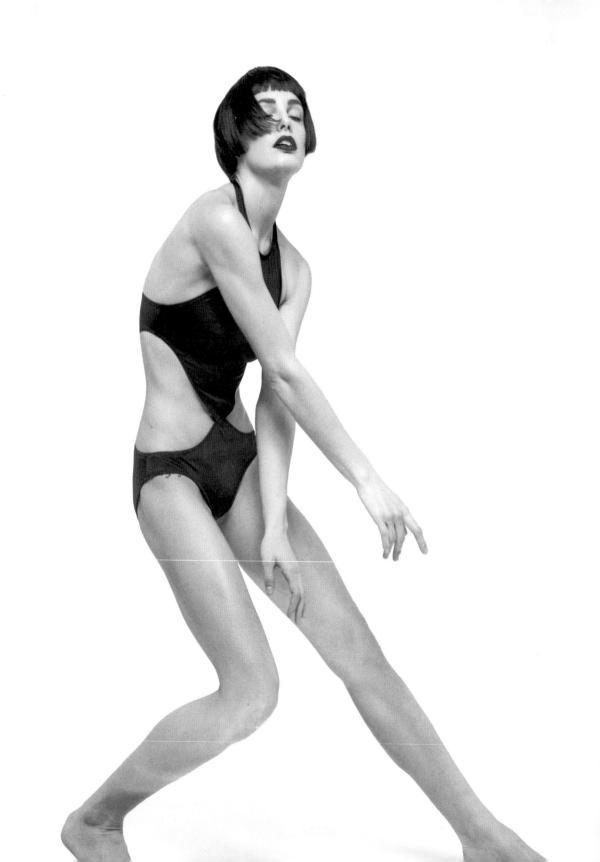

FALL IN LOVE WITH LOVE AGAIN.

UNDERSTAND THE TRUE EXPERIENCE OF UNCONDITIONAL LOVE.

ADOPT A PET.

DOGS TEACH US UNCONDITIONAL LOVE, AND IT IS A LESSON WELL-LEARNED.

MEDITATION
ANYTIME, ANYWHERE

I DON'T ALWAYS HAVE THE OPPORTUNITY TO MEDITATE IN A QUIET, PRIVATE PLACE TO DEAL WITH THE STRESS OF THE DAY, SO I AM HAPPY TO SHARE MY SECRET TO MEDITATING ANYTIME, ANYWHERE:

1 I go to the bathroom, turn out the lights, and close the lid. I sit straight, place my feet hip-width apart, press my shoulders back, lift up from my rib cage, close my eyes, and begin to breathe.

2 I take a minute to focus on my breath and push away all thoughts. **I visualize my breath entering my nostrils and take in waves of pure air in six slow counts,** and release the breath through my mouth in six slow counts with a big *ahhhhh!* You can extend the count to eight and repeat.

3 **Try a five-minute test; the next time, a ten-minute test.** I set a timer on my phone so I don't have to think about how long it's been. Once you are comfortable with the routine, you can increase it to twenty minutes or do two ten-minute sessions.

It works!

DIY
THAI MASSAGE

Massage is incredibly helpful for me mentally and physically, for the perception of my power, and for the strength to work out every day. I was introduced to Thai massages back in the seventies and have been getting them ever since. Similar in philosophy to acupuncture, the application of pressure to specific points on the body opens the flow of energy.

Unlike other types of massage, the Thai modality is not a passive experience: You are stretched; you breathe through it; you are an active participant in the massage.

The combination of active meditation, acupressure, and a good stretch helps me feel totally relaxed, restored, and flexible afterward. A few years ago I met Gilles, a Frenchman who was highly recommended for a great Thai massage. Here is a quick tip from Gilles to help improve flexibility. It's a simple mini-massage you can do at home.

1 SIT CROSS-LEGGED.

2 PLACE YOUR FOREARM PERPENDICULARLY ON YOUR SAME-SIDE QUAD.

3 USE YOUR ULNA BONE (THE UNDERSIDE OF THE FOREARM) TO ROLL OUT ALONG THE INSIDE OF YOUR QUAD, REPEATING, ALL THE WAY UP TO YOUR KNEE.

4 REPEAT OTHER SIDE.

GYROKINESIS
SELF-MASSAGE

GYROKINESIS IS A PRACTICE DEVELOPED BY FORMER DANCER JULIU HORVATH THAT INCREASES FLEXIBILITY, BUILDS OVERALL STRENGTH, AND OPENS ENERGY PATHWAYS THROUGH AN UNINTERRUPTED FLOW OF FOCUSED, RHYTHMIC MOVEMENTS AND COORDINATED BREATHWORK.

CLASSES OFTEN BEGIN WITH A RELAXING SELF-MASSAGE. HERE IS A TOP-TO-TOE TECHNIQUE YOU CAN DO ANYTIME, OR EVEN EVERY DAY WHEN YOU WAKE OR PREPARE FOR BED. THE RHYTHM AND BREATH CREATE AN ACTIVE MEDITATION.

1 Sit up straight on a chair, or preferably a backless stool.

2 Place feet wider than hip-distance apart and sit with straight back. Tilt hips slightly forward to be balanced front, back, and sides.

3 Raise elbows with hands limp at wrists. Start at the top of your head, tapping your fingers, moving around the head and then to the back of the neck and tops of the shoulders.

4 Pull both earlobes down and out, opening your mouth with a wide frowning grimace as you rotate your jaw to open ears. Then pull the outer edges of your ears and continue each action for twelve counts.

5 Next, tap your forehead with your fingertips, same as before, from the center to the sides for twelve counts.

6 Take your thumbs and apply pressure with pulses under your eyebrows at the closest part next to your nose.

7 Use the forefingers of both hands and apply upward pressure to the sinus cavities on either side of the tip of your nose. Again with twelve pulses.

8 Open your mouth with a stretched-wide smile, to a pucker, and then to a wide-open circus smile, again twelve times.

9 Roll your head to one side, gently pulling your head toward your shoulder with your hand to deepen the stretch. Roll your head to facedown, with chin against chest, and then turn your face up, with a count to twelve while breathing throughout. Repeat on opposite side.

THE RITUAL
OF SLEEP

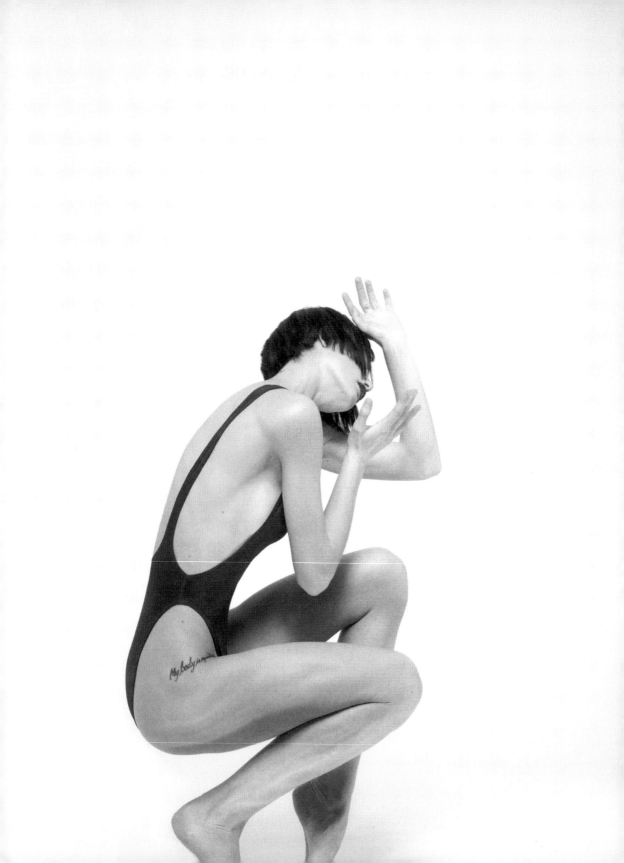

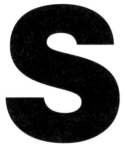leep is the first of the Three Pillars of a healthy lifestyle, and many experts I've spoken to believe it is fifty percent of the pie. To me, it is the best health and beauty secret of all time. Sleep heals. Sleep restores. A good night's sleep makes all the difference for every cell in your body. Sleep is critical for daily restoration. While the body slows down, rests, and resets, the brain is busy, sending signals that trigger healing, repair muscles and tissue, and fight disease. Sleep deprivation is associated with everything from compromised immunity to weight gain and heightened mental health issues.

When I sleep well, I embrace the next day and all of its challenges from a place of calm and control. I feel better. I look better. Most of all, a good night's sleep cleans up all the garbage from the previous day, so I can begin the new day with a good attitude, as an optimist.

I've always treasured sleep. I treat it as something to look forward to, and I approach preparing for bed as a ritual.

From the moment you wake in the morning, everything you do during the day impacts how you will sleep that evening. Therefore it is important to make sure the things you do are complementing a restful night, instead of undermining it.

There have been times when worrying issues have kept me up at night, and I've learned that dealing with anxiety before I go to bed is the key to minimizing the disruption. Be proactive, and chances are you will have more control over the situation, instead of staring at the ceiling, becoming more and more anxious.

For me, meditation breaks, taken as needed throughout the day, have proven to be a great way to temper anything stressful that might throw off my routine. However upsetting the issue, I do all I can to surrender to my breath, and feel the calm wash over my head and shoulders, all the way to my feet. This practice is like exercise: You need to develop the routine, and every day you will get better and better at dispelling the anxiety and fears. If you can do this during the day, and maybe an hour before bedtime, it will be so helpful.

Exercise is an amazing opportunity for sleep preparation, too. In addition to helping naturally reduce stress and anxiety levels, regular exercise has been shown to boost the amount of time the body spends in deep sleep. This is the most physically rejuvenative phase, important for memory and cognitive function. When energy is restored, cells regenerate, and the immune system is strengthened.

If I am feeling on edge after I get home from work and have already exercised earlier in the day, I do a series of calming mat work that puts me right out. Lots of people don't believe in exercise before bed—and it's true, exercise that leaves you energized can interfere with the ability to fall asleep—but I learned this trick several years ago after I had a really ridiculous sleep issue.

I am actually embarrassed to share the story, but here goes:

I was diagnosed with osteoporosis in my forties and have followed many treatment plans over the years. As I was beginning an intensive new protocol, my doctor's assistant instructed me to take the medication in this way: "two A.M., two P.M." I questioned this—*really, take meds every day at two* A.M.?—but she simply insisted that I follow the instructions she had sent via email. So for the next six months I set the clock for a two A.M. wake-up each day, so I could take the medication at the prescribed time. I know I sound foolish even retelling this, but I want good bones, so whatever.

After the six months were up, I visited the doctor. He asked how I was doing, and I said, "Fine. Except now I have a sleep issue, and why do I have to take medication at two in the morning?" He looked at me as if I were nuts, and I felt, yup, ridiculous. He had meant that I should take *two* tablets in the *morning* and *two* tablets at *night*.

But now I had to deal with the issue of waking up daily at two A.M., no alarm needed, and not being able to get back to sleep again, or if I did, not until five A.M. I was groggy and out of sorts in the mornings, and less able to calmly create collections, manage my company, and patiently solve problems. These are key tools for running my business, and having that disruption was not good.

Since my sleep cycle had been reprogrammed, this was far more complicated than adjusting from something like jet lag. I tried everything, with the exception of any type of sleeping pills. Then I developed a routine of active meditation very much like what some folks relate to yoga. And it worked.

EXERCISE IS AN AMAZING OPPORTUNITY FOR SLEEP PREPARATION. IN ADDITION TO HELPING NATURALLY REDUCE STRESS AND ANXIETY LEVELS, REGULAR EXERCISE HAS BEEN SHOWN TO BOOST THE AMOUNT OF TIME THE BODY SPENDS IN DEEP SLEEP.

I've included the detailed steps at the end of this chapter, in NORMA'S GUIDE. It is a routine of rhythmic movements that become hypnotic, exhausting the body and calming the mind. Breathwork is a big part. The reps can be done on a mat on the floor, or in bed. There are times I don't make it to the end and fall asleep, which is why I say try it in bed. I use it on planes (a bit modified, but the concept is the same) and also as a way to get a mat workout while watching TV and relaxing. It may not be for everyone, but I love these steps and practice them when I still feel energetic from the day or am in a different time zone and my body clock is off-kilter.

It's easy to take sleep for granted and to overlook the critical role it plays in health and well-being. This is sacred time planned in a sacred space for the total restoration of every part of our body, for all of the stress it experienced and the work it did during the day. We can't catch up on lost sleep over the weekend, because the body requires each night to repair and refresh. Prioritizing it is a crucial part of aging with power. NK

YOUR BEDROOM IS A SACRED SPACE.

IT SHOULD BE USED JUST FOR SLEEPING OR INTIMATE ENGAGEMENT WITH YOUR PARTNER. IT SHOULD BE CLEAN AND FREE OF ANYTHING NOT CONNECTED WITH SLEEP.

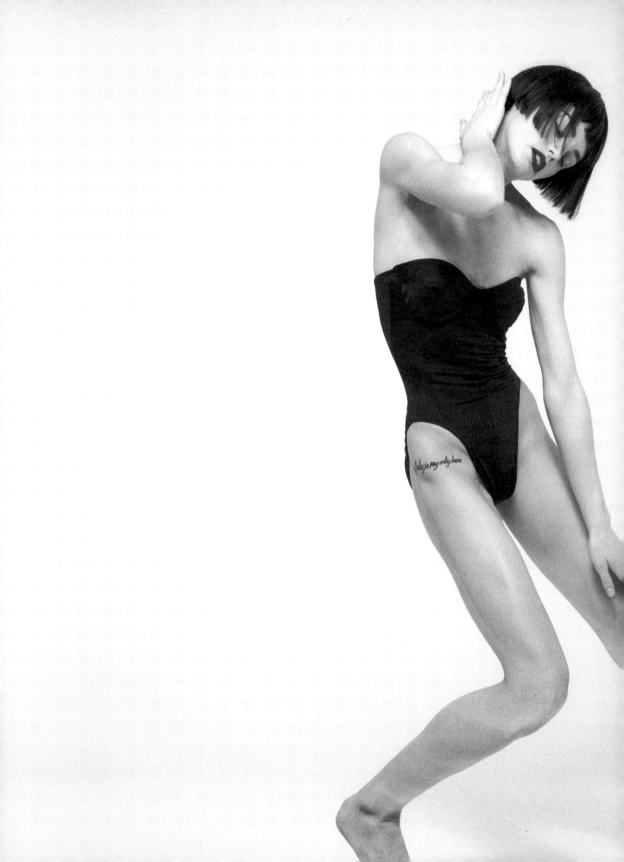

ALWAYS WITHOUT EXCEPTION, YOU MUST MAKE YOUR BED. NEVER GET INTO AN UNMADE BED! EACH NIGHT IS A NEW SPECIAL OPPORTUNITY TO RESTORE AND HEAL FROM THE DAY THAT JUST ENDED.

MAKE YOUR BED AN INVITING AND BEAUTIFUL PLACE TO RESTORE AND RECONNECT.

YOUR BED IS YOUR SANCTUARY.

CAN YOU LIVE WITHOUT A TV IN YOUR BEDROOM?

WATCHING TV, TEXTING, AND EMAILING IN BED REALLY NEED TO BE RETHOUGHT. THESE LIFESTYLE HABITS CAN MAKE A DIFFERENCE IN THE QUALITY OF YOUR SLEEP. BLUE LIGHT EXPOSURE (FROM ALL SCREENS) IN THE EVENING CAN THROW OFF YOUR INTERNAL CLOCK.

GIVE IT A TRY—AVOID THESE STIMULATING ACTIVITIES IN BED.

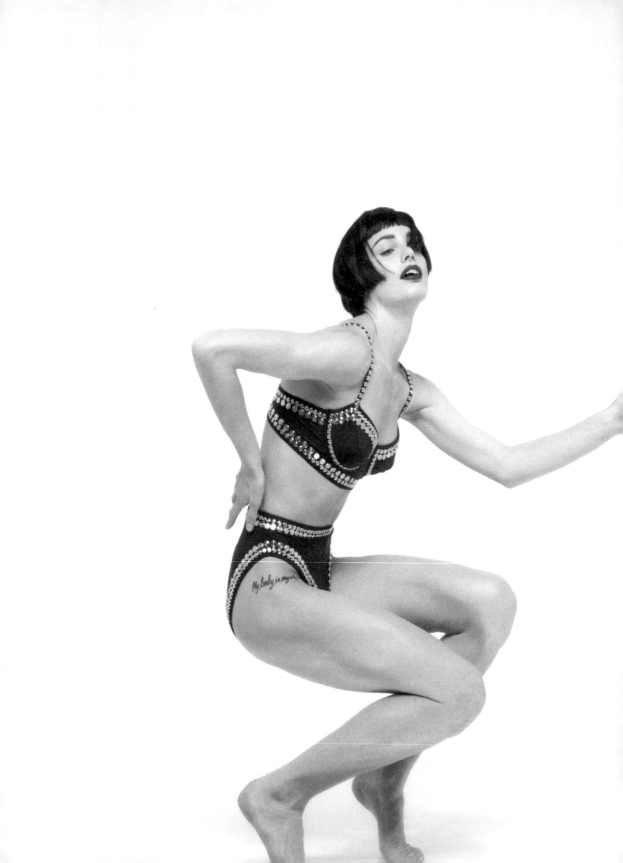

EXERCISE WELCOMES SLEEP AND SLEEP NEEDS EXERCISE.

REGULAR EXERCISE HAS BEEN SHOWN TO IMPROVE SLEEP QUALITY AND DURATION.

I THINK OF IT AS ONE OF THE BEST STRESS REDUCERS IN THE WORLD.

CAFFEINE—IN COFFEE, TEA, EVEN DARK CHOCOLATE—STIMULATES THE NERVOUS SYSTEM AND CAN STAY ELEVATED IN THE BLOOD FOR SIX TO EIGHT HOURS.

YOUR MORNING COFFEE SHOULD BE YOUR LAST OF THE DAY IN ORDER TO COMPLETELY ELIMINATE CAFFEINE FROM YOUR SYSTEM BEFORE SLEEP.

IF YOU NEED A PICK-ME-UP IN THE AFTERNOON, INSTEAD OF CAFFEINE, **TRY MEDITATING!** YES, MEDITATION IS CALMING AND RELAXING, BUT IT ALSO HELPS WITH FOCUS AND CLARITY.

WHAT YOU EAT THROUGHOUT THE DAY CAN AFFECT YOUR SLEEP.

DINNERTIME SHOULD BE TWO TO THREE HOURS BEFORE GOING TO BED.

DINNER SHOULD BE THE SMALLEST AND EASIEST TO DIGEST MEAL OF THE DAY.

IF YOUR DINNER RUNS LATE, TAKE A WALK OUTSIDE OR ON A TREADMILL BEFORE GOING TO SLEEP. LYING DOWN IMMEDIATELY AFTER EATING MAKES PROPER DIGESTION MUCH HARDER.

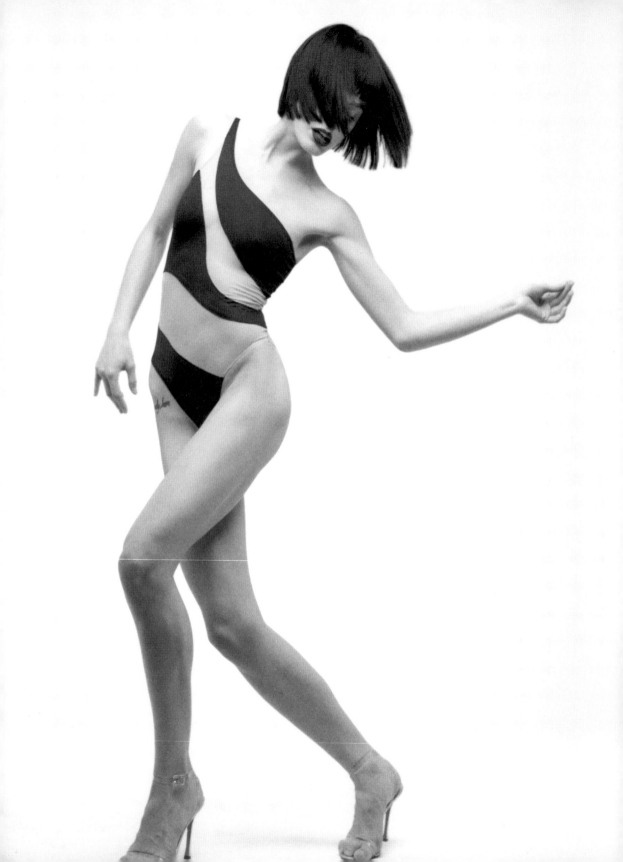

ALCOHOL!

SO MANY PEOPLE LOOK FORWARD TO A DRINK TO RELAX AT THE END OF THE DAY. IT IS A FACT THAT ALCOHOL CAN PUT YOU TO SLEEP, BUT IT MAY ALSO BE THE REASON THAT SLEEP IS SHORT AND UNPRODUCTIVE. IT IS KNOWN TO INCREASE SYMPTOMS OF SLEEP APNEA AND CAN REDUCE MELATONIN PRODUCTION.

I THINK ABOUT HOW FOLKS LOOK AND FEEL WHEN THEY WAKE IN THE MORNING AFTER DRINKING, SHOWING SIGNS THAT ADEQUATE RESTORATION MAY NOT HAVE TAKEN PLACE THE PREVIOUS EVENING.

EVEN WHEN OUT WITH FRIENDS, MIX IN SOME DINNERS WITHOUT A DRINK TO SEE IF THAT IMPROVES YOUR SLEEP.

THINK OF BEDTIME AS A DAILY RITUAL.

HERE ARE MY TIPS TO HELP YOU DESIGN THE SLEEP ENVIRONMENT OF YOUR DREAMS.

1 KEEP YOUR BEDROOM COOL, DARK, AND SMELLING GOOD.

The temperature should be comfortable and a little cooler than the other rooms in your home. Temperatures between sixty and sixty-eight degrees Fahrenheit have been shown to stimulate the production of melatonin, a natural hormone that is essential to the onset of sleep. Body temperature naturally drops as the body anticipates sleep, so a cool room may help you fall asleep faster. Studies show that light inhibits the release of melatonin. A dark bedroom with no light whatsoever is ideal. An eye mask is comfortable and really helps. I believe scent is therapeutic and can be an amazing part of the restorative sleep experience. Scent, from diffusers or essential oils, interacts with our senses to create a tranquil environment. I use a special blend in my diffuser and spray it on my sleep sets each night for an added layer of calm. You may want to consider a humidifier, which adds moisture to the air, or a sound machine, which some studies suggest may help deepen sleep. Both are optional and can be preset to go on and off as needed.

2 INVEST IN YOUR BED.

Your sheets, pillows, and mattress are the most important home furnishings you buy. This is where you purchase the best you can afford and upgrade as soon as you can. A clean bed is so important, so when laundering bedding, use green, unscented products. Choose a mattress density that feels good for you and your mate. Your blanket or comforter must be something where the touch is memorable. My favorite thing is my silk pillowcase. I have other pillows on my bed, but the pillow I actually use for sleep is a standard soft pillow with a white, washable silk pillowcase. I feel like my head is floating on a cloud. Silk against the face is gentle and provides a smooth surface. It causes less friction during the night and has been shown to be better than cotton for both skin and hair. I believe more than anything that a cloud-like pillow with a silk cover is a wonderful sleep enhancer.

3 PREPARE FOR BED.

Don't eat before you go to bed. And minimize how much you drink. By limiting bathroom runs, you reduce the breaks in your sleep and the possible temptation to look at your mobile device and think daytime thoughts, both of which make it more difficult to fall back asleep. While I brush my teeth, wash my face, and moisturize, I am thinking about the last step of letting go of the day. This is a reminder to not take sleep for granted. As I prepare for bed, I choose from a selection of sleep sets I use only for sleep. I do not work out in them, or eat in them, or hang around the house and read in them! I only sleep in them. They are not necessarily expensive; they are special in that I chose them because the fabric, color, and texture all felt perfect for sleeping. Everything feels good on the body, and there is nothing binding or fitted. Your body releases toxins through your skin; the fabric of your sleep clothes should not be compressing.

4 UNPLUG

I have a time each evening when I shut down my devices. It is best to do this at least two hours before you prepare for bed. I have a little sleeping bag I created for my phone. I shut it off, plug it in, and tuck it away. I do not keep it in my bedroom, not even when I travel.

MAP OUT

ACCORDING TO THE NATIONAL SLEEP FOUNDATION, HEALTHY ADULTS REQUIRE SEVEN TO NINE HOURS OF SLEEP EACH NIGHT, BUT WE ALL HAVE DIFFERENT NEEDS. IT'S THE QUALITY OF SLEEP THAT MATTERS AND THAT AFFECTS PHYSICAL AND MENTAL HEALTH.

HOW MANY HOURS OF SLEEP YOU NEED.

IF YOU'RE GETTING ENOUGH SLEEP, YOU SHOULD
FEEL ENERGIZED DURING THE DAY. A REALLY GOOD
WAY TO MONITOR YOUR IDEAL NUMBER OF HOURS
IS TO MAKE NOTE OF THE MORNINGS YOU WAKE UP
WELL RESTED. HOW MANY HOURS DID YOU SLEEP
DURING EACH OF THOSE NIGHTS?

ASSUMING YOU APPROACH EACH NIGHT WITH THE
BEST INTENTIONS—AVOIDING TOO MUCH CAFFEINE,
FOOD, AND DRINK—YOU MIGHT NOTICE THAT AFTER
TWO WEEKS OF A THOUGHTFUL APPROACH TO SLEEP,
SEVEN HOURS DID IT FOR YOU.

IF SEVEN HOURS FEELS RIGHT FOR YOU, IT IS NOW
UP TO YOU TO DETERMINE THE TIME YOU NEED TO GO
TO BED EACH EVENING IN ORDER TO WAKE UP AT THE
APPROPRIATE HOUR THE NEXT DAY. HOWEVER MUCH
SLEEP YOU NEED, KEEP CONSISTENT PATTERNS, EVEN
ON THE WEEKEND. IRREGULAR SLEEP SCHEDULES
CAN ALTER CIRCADIAN RHYTHMS.

NK'S ACTIVE MEDITATION PRE-SLEEP WORKOUT

This is my own sleep solution that I share with friends and that I have found to be helpful. It's something I do every once in a while when I'm having trouble sleeping or still feel stirred up from the day. It puts me right out. I also recommend it for women going through menopause, when, due to hormonal changes, fluctuations in body heat, and the nervous anxiety that goes along with it, it can be hard to feel comfortable in your own skin, never mind in your bed. If it works for you, great; if not, at least you'll get some ab work done. These movements can be done on a mat on the floor by your bed, or in bed. They can be done before going to sleep, or if you wake up in the middle of the night. You can do all three movements in the series, or just focus on one of your choosing. They're simple motions that require you to count and breathe, creating a meditative state. Maintaining focus prevents outside thoughts from cluttering your mind. Every movement is the length of a six-count breath. The sound of each exhalation is important. The number of repetitions exhaust the body, and it's likely you'll fall asleep before you've even finished. A helpful tip is to try it first when you are not in bed or preparing for sleep, just to experience how your body feels and to become familiar with the movements.

Lie flat on your back, arms and legs straight, but relaxed. Position a pillow under your head.

Close your eyes. Breathe in through your nose, hold the breath, and take another short breath; then release with mouth closed and tongue just behind the upper teeth at the roof of your mouth. Repeat the breathing twelve times.

For the first movement:
Turn legs slightly out, hip-distance apart, and lift one leg twelve inches off the bed with the heel facing up. Pause slightly, then slowly bring the leg down and rest before lifting the opposite leg. Alternate legs for fifty to one hundred counts. Keep your abs engaged and concentrate on your breath, exhaling through the nose with closed mouth, following the rhythm of each movement.

For the second movement:
Lift one leg up and over the other leg and tap the mat or bed with your heel. Alternate sides for one hundred repetitions each.

For the third movement:
Bend your knees slightly and place your heels onto the mat or bed. Keep your upper body rested, head still on the pillow and hips in place, and slowly rock your knees side to side gently, only five inches each way. Keep your abs engaged, your breathwork going, and the count at a rhythmic pace. Do one hundred repetitions or more. When you start to feel tired, go further—so if one hundred is not enough, do two hundred. The exhaustion, the breath, and the counting all become your personal lullaby.

YOU
REALLY ARE
WHAT
YOU EAT

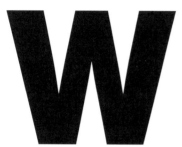

What you eat should be a lifestyle choice, not a fad diet, just like your workouts should be part of your daily routine, and not sporadic. A balanced diet is the second of the Three Pillars for maintaining a healthy life. Food is nutrition, and food is medicine. Knowing which foods fortify the immune system, offer the benefits of healing, and provide high nutritional value, you can easily start filling your cupboard with ingredients that support your mind and body. You will develop a taste for clean, healthy food, making meals and snacks that are delicious and satisfying, and that look beautiful, too.

In my experience, adopting thoughtful eating habits has allowed me to take control of my body and mind and manage the challenges I've faced as I've moved through the decades and the hormonal transitions they bring. Our bodies change constantly from puberty through menopause, and it is important to maintain balance through these ups and downs.

You are not going on a diet; you are adopting a life plan that will become the structure for making the best decisions about how and what you eat.

Here is what I have learned over the years:

Most women have a very complicated relationship with food. When we are unhappy with our bodies, the first thing we often say is that we are "fat" and "need to go on a diet." Our relationship with food can be as toxic as a bad marriage. When we are depressed, we eat bad food; when we are happy and celebrating, we eat bad food; when we don't know what to eat, we tend to eat bad food. We eat huge meals. We eat snacks. And we eat throughout the day without a conscious plan. We eat too much, and for the most part we are not thinking of the consequences bad food has for our mind, body, and

MOST WOMEN HAVE A VERY COMPLICATED RELATIONSHIP WITH FOOD.

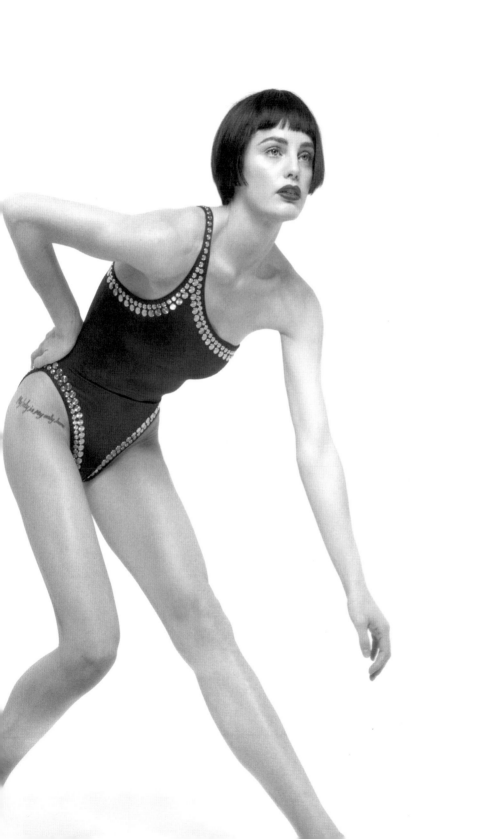

overall health. Even more devastating is the effect on our self-esteem, which reinforces the cycle of poor eating habits. This can be a real setback in terms of our feelings of power and confidence.

Well, this is the time to start taking charge of how you feel about yourself. The more you know about the value of everything you choose to eat and the quantity you need, the happier and healthier you will be.

THE MORE YOU KNOW ABOUT THE VALUE OF EVERYTHING YOU CHOOSE TO EAT, THE HAPPIER AND HEALTHIER YOU WILL BE.

LISTEN TO YOUR BODY

My personal relationship with food began as a teenager when I realized that how awful I felt after I ate was directly related to the type of food I was eating and how my body was digesting it. I don't think it ever occurred to my parents that some of the things I ate—dairy, red meat—could be the cause of my ongoing stomach pain. Everyone ate everything back then. No one said they were lactose-intolerant or vegetarian. There was no conversation about food allergies, and there were no resources available to help me find better choices. All of that was totally unheard-of when I was growing up.

During the eighties I started doing my own research and worked on changing my diet. I eliminated meat altogether and started eating plant-based. I fell back on the simple salads I'd always loved—dressed with olive oil and lemon—and began learning about the nutritional benefits of nuts, beans, mushrooms, green vegetables, and colorful foods. I was traveling a lot for my licenses during this time, most frequently to Japan. I immediately fell in love with Japanese food: always fresh, dairy-free, no fast food (at the time), and green tea! This became my base. Eating this way made me feel so good. There was a small Japanese restaurant on Fifty-Sixth Street near my company headquarters in New York, and I was there every day for lunch and dinner until 2012, when it closed. On the restaurant's second floor, they offered private dinners and karaoke. After presenting a collection, my team and I would go to eat and sing through the night!

Listening to your body and what works for you is super important. When you suspect a food type is making you feel off, try eliminating it from your diet for two weeks. If you don't see results right away, keep trying the elimination technique until you identify the foods that are creating distress.

HOW MUCH WE EAT, AND WHEN

From my twenties on, I was aware of my weight. With fashion being so dominant in my life, how clothes fit was always important. Until I became fully informed about the food we eat and how it is produced, I just followed the latest fad. Crazy diets, or just not eating, was the norm.

The simple secret I've learned is that if we eat quality food we will feel fulfilled and less controlled by our cravings. The amount of food we need is much less than you might imagine. Portion size counts. By eating less, we can focus on making each meal or snack one that will benefit our overall well-being. Shop for healthy foods and think about the size of the portions and the density of the nutritious value in each meal, and you will be surprised how easy it is to feel satisfied after eating.

Intermittent fasting can be helpful for many reasons. First and foremost, it gives your digestive system a break and helps rid the body of toxins. It imposes a natural cleanse, which I find energizing and uplifting. I have experimented with fasting since my thirties, and with proper guidance, I learned how to healthily cleanse my system and help manage my weight this way.

Intermittent fasting offers many easy-to-follow variations (see my tips in NORMA'S GUIDE, page 110). What I really like about a fasting schedule is that it creates structure for thoughtful food planning and behavior. Mapping out what you will eat before and after you break your fast is part of the program, so you focus on making quality choices.

LISTENING TO YOUR BODY AND WHAT WORKS FOR YOU IS SUPER IMPORTANT.

FOOD AS LOVE

Self-love is a theme in this book that is very much a part of the healthy lifestyle protocol. What we choose to eat is an indication of how we feel about ourselves. If we realize we are eating too much, especially of the wrong food choices and at midnight, the sirens should go off, saying, *Whoa, you need some lovin'*. The most important way to receive that love is by first giving it to yourself.

Food can heal. It can make you look amazing. It can be something you share with people you love, especially if it will make everyone healthier and happier. Think long and hard before you plan a meal. Show the people in your life some love, and do it through food.

YOUR BODY
WORKS HARD
TO ABSORB
WHAT YOU
PUT IN IT,
SO GIVE IT
THE BEST.

Also give gifts of food to those you love. I send bottles of olive oil from my favorite orchards in the olive belt of France and Spain to my friends for the holidays, just after the new harvest. It tastes great, and the benefits are plentiful.

My relationship with food and proper nutrition has become a great comfort for helping me to stay healthy and sustain the proper weight for my body. Wholesome food—the fewer ingredients in a dish and the less sauce, the better—is my formula. Your body works hard to absorb what you put in it, so give it the best.

It can be especially difficult to maintain a perfect lifestyle and stay on track when hormones are affecting your emotional well-being. The most important way to balance excess is to limit the number of days you go off a healthy plan. The important thing to remember is that heading back to a thoughtful diet puts the power back in your control.

Eat good food, eat real food, and eat it in controlled portions. Feel better, look better, and teach your children the joy of how delicious healthy food can be without excessive amounts of sugar, salt, and poor fats. Make it your lifestyle. The results will empower you. NK

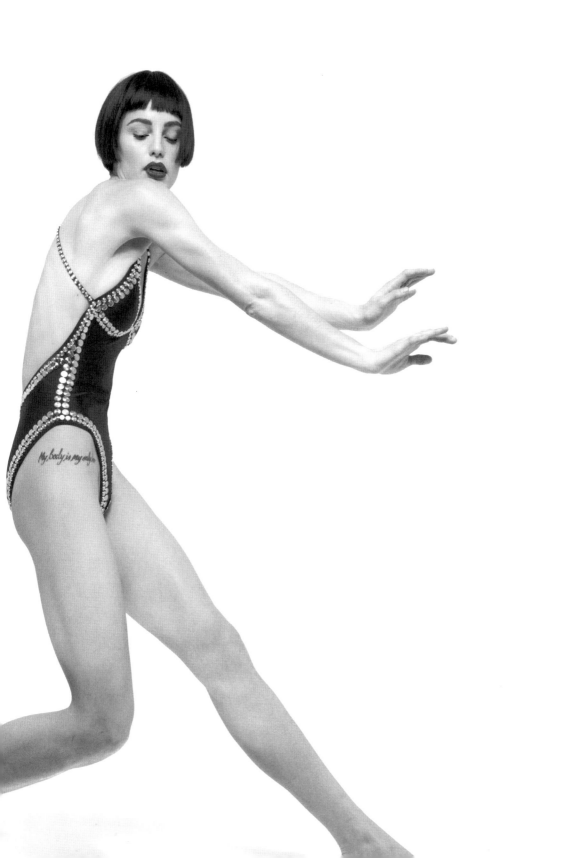

"LET FOOD BE YOUR MEDICINE AND MEDICINE BE YOUR FOOD."

—HIPPOCRATES

MAINTAINING A HEALTHY IMMUNE SYSTEM IS A PROACTIVE APPROACH TO YOUR PERSONAL HEALTH CARE.

POSITIVE LIFESTYLE CHANGES THAT YOU CAN MAKE YOURSELF HELP ENSURE FEWER DOCTOR VISITS.

START WITH A DIET INCREASING THE INTAKE OF NUTRIENT-RICH FOODS.

FOR OPTIMAL HEALTH, ELIMINATE PROCESSED FOODS WITH SUGAR AND SALT ADDITIVES AS WELL AS CHEMICALS, HORMONES, AND PRESERVATIVES.

YOU CAN VISIT A NUTRITIONIST TO HELP DEVISE A HEALTHY PLAN THAT WORKS FOR YOU.

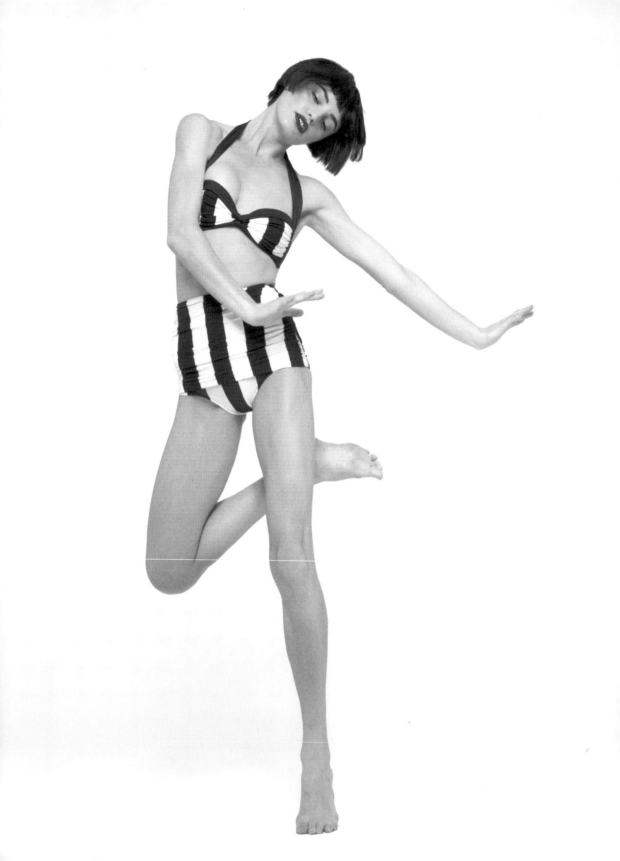

EAT A PLANT BASED DIET.

DR. ANDREW WEIL TAUGHT ME THAT OUR IMMUNE SYSTEM MUST BE FUELED IN ORDER TO KEEP US HEALTHY.

SINCE I STARTED EATING PLANT-BASED, NEARLY FORTY YEARS AGO, I'VE SEEN A REAL DIFFERENCE IN HOW I FEEL.

PLANT-BASED DIETS RICH IN FRUITS, VEGETABLES, GRAINS, LEGUMES, NUTS, AND SEEDS ARE FILLED WITH ANTI-INFLAMMATORY AND ANTIOXIDANT-PACKED VITAMINS AND MINERALS. HEART-HEALTHY FOODS EMPHASIZING FRESH, WHOLE INGREDIENTS HAVE BEEN SHOWN TO HELP REDUCE THE RISK OF DIABETES AND CERTAIN CANCERS, AND SLOW OR PREVENT COGNITIVE DECLINE.

GET ALL THE HELP YOU CAN FROM GOOD FOOD TO KEEP YOU HEALTHY AND LOOKING GOOD.

IT IS A FACT...

THAT EATING
A PLANT-BASED
DIET AND
BUYING LOCALLY
PRODUCED FOOD
HAVE A SMALLER
ENVIRONMENTAL
FOOTPRINT.

IT'S GOOD FOR THE PLANET AND GOOD FOR YOU.

MAKE SURE THE FOOD YOU EAT IS COLORFUL.

DARK RED AND GREEN VEGETABLES AND FRUITS ENSURE POWERFUL VITAMIN INTAKE.

GMO TECHNOLOGY IS NOT IN HARMONY WITH HUMAN BIOLOGY.

FROM CAVEMAN TIMES UNTIL NOW, WE HAVE BEEN MEANT TO CONSUME CELL BIOLOGY AS NATURE PLANNED.

THE CONSEQUENCES OF FOODS ENGINEERED WITH **GMOS** (GENETICALLY MODIFIED ORGANISMS) ARE NOT FULLY KNOWN; HOWEVER, THERE IS ENOUGH INFORMATION THAT IT SHOULD SIGNAL CONCERN.

LEARN MORE ABOUT THE FOOD YOU BUY.

A GREEN JUICE WITH LEMON, OLIVE OIL, AND
A DASH OF PINK SEA SALT IS A GREAT TWIST ON
REGULAR GREEN JUICES.

DRINK YOUR SALAD

WHEN HEALTHY FOODS ARE DELICIOUS, IT IS SO
EASY TO MAKE THEM PART OF YOUR LIFESTYLE.

POWDERED GREENS IN COCONUT WATER
OR AS SUPPLEMENTS ARE A MUST IF YOU
ARE MISSING OUT ON VEGETABLES. PERFECT
FOR TRAVEL WHEN YOU ARE NOT SURE WHERE
YOU WILL GET YOUR GREENS.

DON'T EAT SUGAR EVER

YOU REALLY ARE WHAT YOU EAT

I BELIEVE **SUGAR IS BAD.** PLAIN AND SIMPLE.

IN ITS NATURAL FORM, IN FRUITS AND VEGETABLES, SUGAR IS HEALTHY IN MODERATION, BUT ADDED IN EXCESS TO PACKAGED FOODS, REFINED SUGAR HAS BEEN LINKED TO A HEIGHTENED RISK OF CHRONIC HEALTH ISSUES, FROM OBESITY AND TYPE 2 DIABETES TO HEART DISEASE AND SOME CANCERS.

IT DOESN'T DO YOUR COMPLEXION ANY FAVORS, EITHER. A DOCTOR ONCE DESCRIBED SUGAR'S OXIDIZING EFFECT ON CELLS TO ME AS AKIN TO "RUST." THE RUST STARTS TO DECAY AND AGE THE CELL. THIS ACCELERATED CELLULAR AGING ALSO HARMS THE BUILDING BLOCKS OF COLLAGEN AND ELASTIN, CAUSING SKIN TO SAG PREMATURELY.

SUGAR IS ADDED TO SO MANY PACKAGED FOODS, AND WHEN WE EAT IT, WE CRAVE MORE, OFTEN NOT THINKING ABOUT THE HARM IT CAN CAUSE OUR BODY, MIND, AND BEHAVIOR. THE SUGAR RUSH IS WELL-KNOWN. IT IS SHORT-LIVED AND CAN END IN LOW ENERGY AND CREATE NEGATIVE BEHAVIOR. JUST WITNESS A CHILD AFTER EATING CANDY TO SEE WHAT HAPPENS TO ALL OF US. IT IS NEVER TOO LATE TO MONITOR THE SUGAR IN YOUR LIFE.

WHEN I FOLLOW AN ALKALINE
DIET, I FEEL CLEANER AND BETTER.
I CAN FEEL THE DIFFERENCE.

THE BODY WORKS HARD TO MAINTAIN A HEALTHY
INTERNAL PH, BUT STRESS AND CERTAIN
FOODS CAN THROW OFF THE BALANCE, CREATING
AN ACIDIC ENVIRONMENT THAT CHALLENGES
THE IMMUNE SYSTEM AND CAN HAVE A NEGATIVE
IMPACT ON OVERALL HEALTH.

NEUTRALIZE YOUR SYSTEM WITH ALKALINE FOODS AND AN ALKALINE LIFESTYLE.

CREATE MEALS BASED ON ALKALIZING
FOODS LIKE FRUITS, VEGETABLES,
NUTS, AND LEGUMES, WHICH DO NOT
INTRODUCE MORE ACIDITY INTO
YOUR SYSTEM.

IF YOU EAT MEAT, MAKE IT ORGANIC AND GRASS-FED

WHICH IS FREE OF HORMONES, ANTIBIOTICS, AND PESTICIDES.

AND I ADVISE KEEPING IT TO A LIMITED AMOUNT.

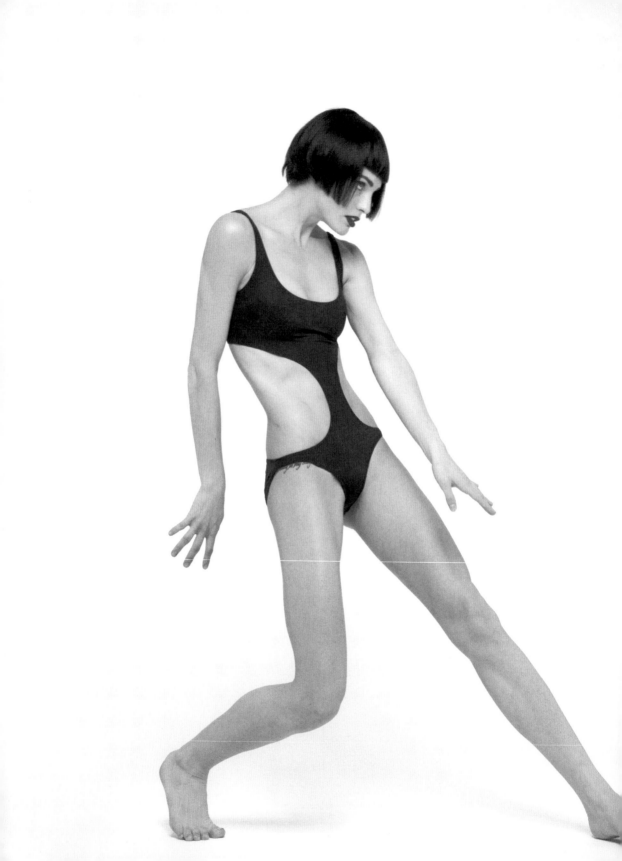

DON'T ALLOW SODA IN YOUR HOME.

KEEP IT AWAY FROM THOSE YOU LOVE.

THE AMOUNT OF SUGAR IN MOST SODAS IS EXCESSIVE, AND TOO MUCH SUGAR IS BAD FOR YOU.

WEAR A BIKINI IN THE WINTER WHILE COOKING

AS A GREAT JUDGMENT
CHECK ON FOOD
CHOICES WHEN WE ARE
SPENDING MORE TIME
INDOORS IN WARM,
LAYERED CLOTHES.

A HEALTHY GUT IS IMPORTANT FOR GOOD HEALTH.

BACTERIA IN THE DIGESTIVE TRACT IS A FACT OF LIFE.

BALANCE THE GOOD AND BAD BACTERIA TO SUPPORT A POWERFUL IMMUNE SYSTEM AND TO AID DIGESTION.

PROBIOTICS — FROM HEALTHY FOOD SOURCES AND SUPPLEMENTS — HELP ACHIEVE EQUILIBRIUM.

TAKE TWO TABLESPOONS OF

RECENT STUDIES HAVE SHOWN THAT TART CHERRIES ARE AN ANTI-INFLAMMATORY SUPERFRUIT WITH MANY GREAT BENEFITS.

TART CHERRY

CHECK OUT THIS LIST:
- PLENTIFUL SOURCE OF VITAMINS, ANTIOXIDANTS, AND POLYPHENOLS
- IMMUNE SYSTEM BOOSTER
- SHOWN TO HELP INCREASE MUSCLE STRENGTH AND TO SPEED RECOVERY AFTER PHYSICAL ACTIVITY AND REDUCE JOINT PAIN
- RICH IN MELATONIN, WHICH CAN IMPROVE SLEEP QUALITY
- MAY REDUCE HEADACHE AND MIGRAINE PAIN

CONCENTRATE A DAY.

ALCOHOL IS UNDER SCRUTINY, ESPECIALLY WHEN IT COMES TO HEALTH ISSUES FOR WOMEN. ALCOHOL IS KNOWN TO AFFECT SLEEP, WHICH IMPACTS HOW YOU FEEL AND HOW YOU LOOK. IT IS HIGH ON THE LIST OF INFLAMMATORIES, ALONG WITH SMOKING. IT IS FULL OF SUGAR, AND NEW RESEARCH SUGGESTS THAT IT MAY HEIGHTEN THE RISK OF BREAST CANCER AND ITS RECURRENCE.

DRINK LESS ALCOHOL.

A WOMAN'S SIZE AND LEVEL OF HYDRATION PLAY A BIG ROLE IN HOW QUICKLY THE EFFECTS OF ALCOHOL IMPACT BEHAVIOR. WE NEED TO BE RESPONSIBLE FOR KNOWING WHAT WE CAN PHYSICALLY HANDLE. INEXPERIENCE CAN LEAVE YOU VULNERABLE. IT WORKS IN YOUR FAVOR TO BE IN CHARGE IN SOCIAL SITUATIONS.

I OFTEN THINK THAT WHEN PEOPLE FEEL, AND QUITE FRANKLY LOOK, AWFUL THE MORNING AFTER DRINKING, THIS SHOULD BE A SIGN THAT THERE ARE ISSUES WHEN ALCOHOL IS CONSUMED. HOW MUCH MORE DO WE NEED TO KNOW IN ORDER TO FIND ANOTHER RELAXING SUBSTITUTE?

IF YOU DON'T DRINK COFFEE...

DON'T START.

I USED TO DRINK TEN CUPS A DAY.
WHEN I STOPPED, I FELT CALM AND
BALANCED. I REALIZED THE EFFECT
COFFEE WAS HAVING ON ME.

CAFFEINE CAN CERTAINLY KEEP YOU
GOING, BUT IT'S NOT NECESSARILY
THE BEST THING FOR YOUR NERVOUS
SYSTEM, OR FOR YOUR SLEEP.

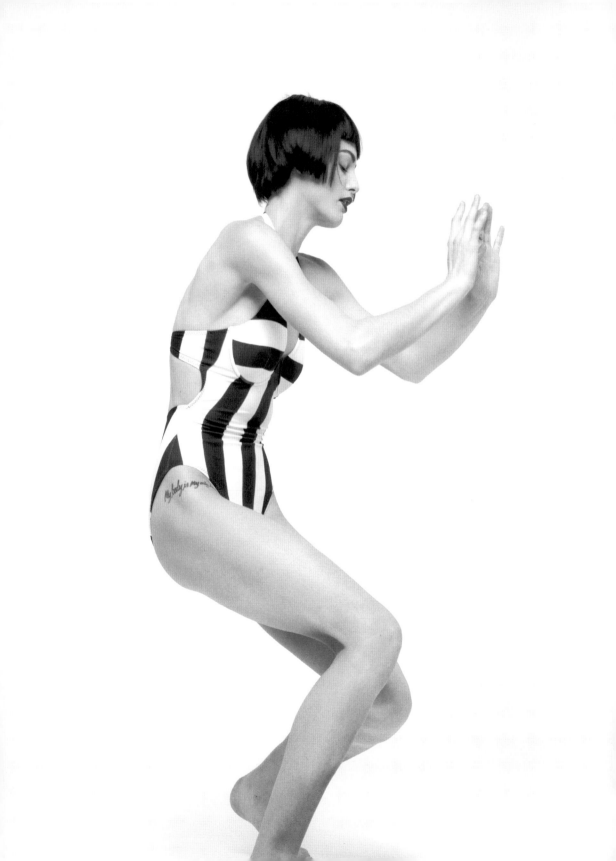

ENZYMES...

ARE A PART OF THE DIGESTIVE PROCESS.

SUPPLEMENTING ENZYMES AS
THEY NATURALLY DECREASE WITH AGE
AIDS NUTRIENT ABSORPTION.

FOR THOSE WHO EXPERIENCE
BLOATING, ESPECIALLY FROM
LACTOSE INTOLERANCE,
AN OVER-THE-COUNTER LACTASE
SUPPLEMENT IS HELPFUL FOR EASING
DISCOMFORT WHEN EATING DAIRY.

YOU REALLY ARE WHAT YOU EAT

HEAVY METALS, WHICH ARE TOXIC IN ELEVATED QUANTITIES, CAN AFFECT YOUR HEALTH AND OVERALL WELL-BEING.

SUBSTITUTE

- PLASTIC BOTTLES WITH GLASS
- ALUMINUM PANS WITH CAST-IRON SKILLETS
- CANNED FOODS WITH FROZEN OR VACUUM-PACKED FRUITS, VEGETABLES, AND LEGUMES

CHOOSE SMALL, WILD FRESH FISH OVER LARGER AND BOTTOM-FEEDING FISH, WHICH CONSUME HIGH LEVELS OF MERCURY.

REDUCE THE METALS IN YOUR BODY.

INCORPORATE POWDERED GREENS AND SELECTED CHLORELLA (NUTRIENT-DENSE ALGAE) INTO YOUR DIET TO HELP CLEAR METALS AND OTHER TOXINS FROM YOUR SYSTEM.

KNOW YOUR BODY AND TAKE ACTION TO PREVENT MALFUNCTION.

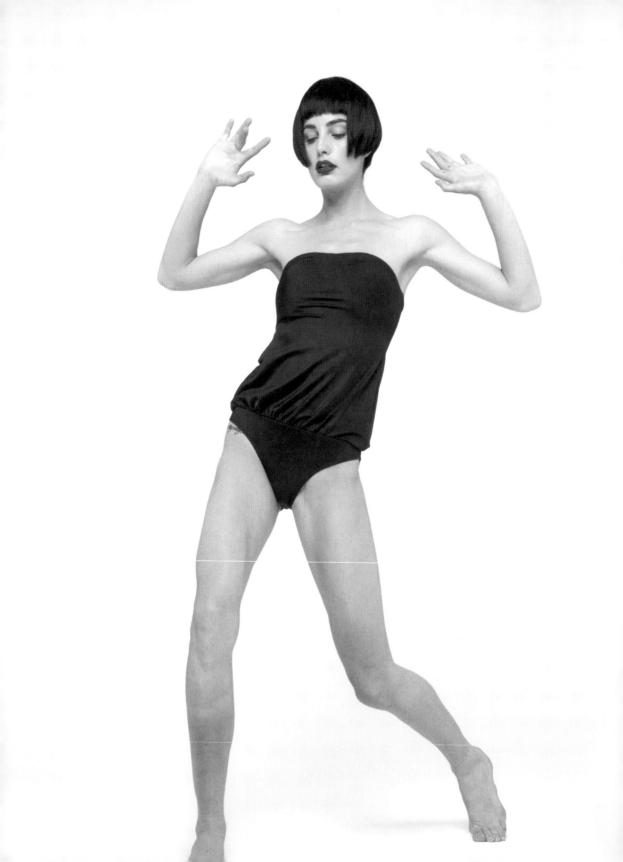

DRINK PLENTY OF WATER.

- ADD LEMON, ONE OF THE BEST ALKALINE FOODS ONCE METABOLIZED, AND GINGER TO CALM DIGESTION AND TO NATURALLY DEBLOAT!
- THE WATER IN GREEN JUICES—SANS THE FRUIT—IS THE PUREST WATER. ENJOY THE FRESHNESS AND NUTRITIONAL BENEFIT OF GREEN JUICE WHILE HYDRATING WITH THE BEST WATER.
- TRY ALKALINE WATER FILTERS FOR ANOTHER PURE WATER OPTION.

YOUR HOME IS
YOUR SAFE PLACE
ONLY STOCK FOOD
THAT WILL MAKE YOU
FEEL GOOD AND LOOK GOOD

GO TO YOUR KITCHEN AND GET A BIG TRASH BAG.

1 Throw away anything that has sugar or is a packaged cracker, a chip … You know what I mean!

2 Sodas, flavored teas, and other beverages with sugars—throw them out! Do it now!

3 Throw out the ketchup, mustard, mayo—all the packaged condiments and dressings.

4 Cereals—throw them out unless they contain no sugar and are organic.

5 Dairy, eggs, meat, and poultry are often subject to antibiotics and hormones. Fruits and vegetables are subject to pesticides.
Knowing where your food was grown or raised is really important.
Make sure it is organic and hormone-free.

NOW GET THE FOLLOWING:

1 **Olive oil**, **lemons**, **sea salt**, and **turmeric**: My favorite dressing for salads and over raw or steamed vegetables. Olive oil has countless uses and benefits from cleansing the liver to lubricating the body and keeping you regular.

2 **Ginger**: Great for digestion. I always have ginger and lemons on hand for hot and cold drinks.

3 **Nuts** and **berries**—especially blueberries, because they have the least amount of sugar.

4 Have plenty of **water** in the house; filtered is great.

5 Go to the organic market and get seasonal local produce and **fresh greens** of any kind. Include **colorful vegetables** and **low-sugar fruits**. Flash-freezing is a way to keep produce like **berries** and **greens** fresh longer and at your fingertips for smoothies.

6 **Powdered greens**: A good source of calcium for bone health.

7 **Avocados**: Loaded with nutrients, healthy fat, and fiber. Keep them in the fridge so they stay fresh longer.

8 **Yams**: Packed with nutrition and fiber.

9 **Lentils** and **chickpeas**: Great sources of protein and essential nutrients.

10 **Fatty fish**: High in omega-3s.

11 **Coconut-based yogurt**: Full of antioxidants and probiotics.

12 **Sardines**: Heart-healthy and calcium- and mineral-rich.

MY RECIPES

NOW YOU HAVE A GOOD START FOR DEVELOPING RECIPES WITH INGREDIENTS THAT WILL MAKE YOU WELL. IN THE SUMMER, I LOVE TO MAKE COLD SOUPS AND SALADS FILLED WITH BEANS, NUTS, AND FRUIT. SOUPS OF PURÉED VEGETABLES OR STEAMED VEGGIES IN BROTH WITH LEMON AND GINGER ARE NOURISHING COMFORT FOOD IN THE WINTER. ANOTHER HEARTY WINTER DISH I LOVE IS BEANS, STEAMED SQUASH, CARROTS, BROCCOLI, AND SPINACH OVER BROWN RICE. HERE ARE MORE OF MY FAVORITE RECIPES, WHICH ARE SO MUCH FUN TO MAKE AND CREATE:

WALNUT AND BLUEBERRY SNACK

One of my favorite snacks is blueberries and walnuts, both of which have been shown to be good for breast health. They are a great combo that I believe are as good as medicine and should be enjoyed by all women. I often eat frozen berries as a dessert or a snack. They are delicious in the summer, cooling and crunchy. They melt very quickly and can be blended into smoothies. My favorite smoothie combines **blueberries** and **walnuts** with **gluten-free oat** or **almond milk**.

P.S. FLASH-FREEZING RIPE FRUIT, WHEN IT IS JUST-PICKED AND MOST NUTRITIOUS, HAS BEEN SHOWN TO RETAIN NUTRIENTS BETTER.

**NORMA'S
GUIDE**
YOU
REALLY ARE
WHAT
YOU EAT

OLIVE OIL POPCORN

You will never be able to eat movie popcorn again!

1 Cover the bottom of a saucepan with a quarter inch of **olive oil**.

2 Add **organic kernels**, shake to make sure all are covered, and pop over medium-high heat.

3 In a large bowl, drizzle popcorn with more **olive oil**, to your taste.

4 Sprinkle with **sea salt**. (My favorite is Real Salt from Utah. It is said to be the cleanest salt in the world.)

5 Feel free to add **spices** of your choice!

TURMERIC DRESSING

Help reduce inflammation with turmeric! "Inflammation" refers to your body's process of fighting things that harm it. When something damages your cells, the body releases chemicals that trigger a response from your immune system. The process lasts a few hours, or days in the case of acute inflammation like infection or injury, as the body heals and restores normal tissue function. Turmeric is a spice that has been used as a medicinal herb in India for thousands of years. It contains the compound curcumin, which is believed to be a powerful anti-inflammatory and antioxidant. It has been linked to increased brain function and may be helpful in treating depression. Here is a delicious suggestion for how to incorporate turmeric into your diet. I recommend trying this dressing, with its beautiful golden color, on everything:

Olive oil   **Sprinkle of sea salt**

Lemon   **Generous amount of tumeric**

It is so delicious you can try it over steamed or raw vegetables. My favorite is with raw cauliflower. I munch on this all day, and a day later it tastes even better, so I tend to make a big bowl and put it in the fridge.

PURÉED YAM SOUP

I love this recipe because it is a three-in-one: It can be a warm puréed soup, a pudding, or an ice cream. Yes! There are so many yams in so many different colors, from pale pink to purple! From a creative, visual standpoint, you can imagine the fun in using a few at the same time, and layering them as a pudding. Yams fit perfectly into the idea of food as medicine for women, especially, since they may ease symptoms of menopause as well as help reduce inflammation, control blood sugar, and improve digestive health and cholesterol levels. It's all about healing foods and color!

AS A SOUP

1 Scoop a cooked **yam** or two or three into a blender.

2 Add **gluten-free oat** or **almond milk** for desired consistency—as thick or thin as you prefer.

3 You can add unflavored **nutritional powders**, which will also add thickness, so keep this in mind.

4 Heat if desired, or pour into bowls.

5 Add a handful of **frozen blueberries** and chopped **walnuts** for garnish.

AS A PUDDING

1 Adjust the liquid so the purée takes on a pudding consistency.

2 I love pouring this into a tall, clear glass and adding layers of pudding, **blueberries**, and ground or chopped **walnuts** to create a parfait.

3 Chill in the fridge.

AS ICE CREAM

1 The purée can be either the same consistency as or thicker than the pudding. You can add ground **nuts** when blending the purée. You will not need to add anything sweet to most yams, but I have added **manuka honey** for friends.

2 Place in a freezable cup or container and freeze.

**NORMA'S
GUIDE
YOU
REALLY ARE
WHAT
YOU EAT**

SQUASH BREAKFAST PORRIDGE

I love something warm to break the fast. Squash is perfect for this.

1 Scoop a cooked or baked **acorn squash** into a blender and add **oat** or **almond milk**.

2 You can add **nutritional powders** that are flavorless, like collagen powder, as well. This will thicken the purée and make it more like a pudding.

3 Heat up, if desired.

4 Add a sprinkle of **cinnamon**.

5 For more texture and some crunch, add chopped **nuts** and **raisins**.

MY BONE-HEALTH SMOOTHIE

Because I have bone issues, and am lactose intolerant, I am constantly searching for new, dairy-free ways to absorb as much calcium as I can through food in order to complement the supplements and treatment I take. Since I started this smoothie routine—a super-delicious and healthy green drink—I have seen an improvement in my bone-density tests. We all absorb nutrients differently. For me, this works.

1 I fill my large blender tightly with greens—a combination of **kale**, **collards**, and **spinach**—halfway, then add a small **avocado** and **green powders**.

2 I add unflavored **collagen powders** (good for skin, hair, and nails), a handful of **blueberries** or **blackberries**, and water, and blend.

3 I like the smoothie to have the consistency of a purée; sometimes I eat it with a spoon, and, of course, with some **nuts**.

4 You can add **olive oil**, as well, and **sea salt**, if you leave out the berries.

P.S. I BUY EXTRA KALE, COLLARD GREENS, AND SPINACH AND PUT THEM IN THE FREEZER IMMEDIATELY SO I HAVE FROZEN GREENS READY ANYTIME.

NUT AND SEED . . . BREAD

The bread that will make you feel good, is good for you, and will keep you regular.

Bread has always been a great love of mine, especially because of my olive oil obsession. The problem is traditional breads are not a good source of nutrition. This, my favorite bread of all time, is actually good for you and tastes good, too! I discovered it when visiting a friend in the Caribbean. There was a bakery we would go to, drawn in by the delicious scent. There was always a small loaf of bread coming out of the oven. I so much wanted to taste the bread, and was trying to remain strong, until I heard the baker say that it was a bread made without flour, just with seeds and nuts: a super-healthy bread that, as a side benefit, kept you regular! Okay, so obsessed, totally obsessed, I begged for the recipe. I am not and have never been a baker, because my diet has been primarily plant-based, but my oven, which remains lonely most of the time, has been turning out this nut-and-seed bread ever since. I like to bake several loaves at a time, then slice and freeze them for ready-to-eat use once popped in the toaster. Add avocado, olive oil, or manuka honey, and you will have a nutritious taste sensation for breakfast, lunch, or dinner. This is also a fantastic home-baked gift for friends and family!

1 cup sunflower seeds

½ cup pumpkin seeds

½ cup flax seeds

½ cup almonds

1½ cups rolled oats

2 tablespoons chia seeds

4 tablespoons psyllium seed husks
 (3 tablespoons if using powder)

1 tablespoon fine-grain sea salt

3 tablespoons melted coconut oil

1½ cups water

**NORMA'S
GUIDE**
YOU
REALLY ARE
WHAT
YOU EAT

1 Pour all dry ingredients into a loaf pan and stir well.

2 Whisk together oil and water and add to the dry ingredients. Mix well until everything is completely soaked and the dough becomes thick but manageable (add one or two teaspoons of water as needed).

3 Smooth out the top with the back of a spoon.

4 Let the dough sit on the counter uncovered for two hours or more, until it retains its shape when pulled away from the sides of the pan.

5 Preheat oven to 350°F/175°C.

6 Place loaf pan on the middle rack and bake for 20 minutes.

7 Remove the bread from the pan; place it upside down on the rack and bake for another 30 to 40 minutes.

8 The bread is done when it makes a hollow sound when tapped with a spoon.

9 Let cool completely before slicing.

CONSIDER QUALITY SUPPLEMENTS.

Fresh whole food is always the best source of vitamins and minerals, but depending on our dietary habits and health history, sometimes we could all use a little backup. Everyone's needs are different, and it is important to make sure any supplements you are taking work well together—a good thing to discuss with your doctor.

Here is a look at my daily regimen for overall well-being:

- **CALCIUM**, for bone health

- **VITAMIN D$_3$**, which supports calcium absorption

- **VITAMIN C**, for bone health and immunity

- **MAGNESIUM**, for regularity and strong bones

- **RED YEAST RICE WITH CoQ10**, for cholesterol control

- **CURCUMIN**, from turmeric, for joint health and reducing inflammation

- **OLIVE OIL**, a teaspoon a day, at least, for regularity and reducing inflammation

INTERMITTENT FASTING.
SO EASY.

Intermittent fasting is worth trying to see if it suits your lifestyle. I find that these periodic cleanses benefit my body, mind, and soul, especially when mixed with sleep, yoga, and meditation. Fasts can be practiced weekly, monthly, quarterly, or any time that fits your schedule. (If you plan to try fasting, please speak to your doctor first, especially if you are on any medication.) Fasts don't have to be events that interrupt your life. Those never work. The idea is to do something healthy you can maintain. For me, fasting has become part of the way I live. The long-term effect is that your body gets used to having a nice long break. When you eat again, it has had some time off, which helps you digest food better. It's not a painful experience; it's something I feel good about doing, and I feel lighter afterward. Once you complete a fast, the desire for healthy food increases, and the desire for large quantities of food decreases. I eat better meals because I plan them carefully and focus on the quality of the food I'm eating. What makes fasting easy is that you have a clear start time and end time. I have done fasts from twenty-four to thirty-six hours a week. Here's a great one for beginners that I do all the time.

SIXTEEN-HOUR FAST

I practice a sixteen-hour fast several days a week. On this schedule, during which eight of the hours are my sleep or rest time, I basically eat two meals a day, and it works for me.

It starts after my last meal of the day, which for me is typically eight P.M. This means that noon the following day is when I break the fast. Until then, I drink liquids. When I wake in the morning, at five-thirty each day, I have tea, or a non-caffeinated coffee alternative like cardamom coffee, made from the spice, or mushroom coffee, a super-healthy drink made from dried mushrooms. Around nine-thirty, I might have some warm water with ginger and lemon.

The meal before the fast and the meal to break the fast are important. The fewer choices you have for when to eat, the more thought you will put into what you eat. What you eat should have value and how much you eat should match your desired healthy body mass. The old-school food measure used to be that two fists are the size of the amount of food you should eat at each meal. This is truly just a way to say quality far exceeds quantity.

After the cleanse, transition to small portions of easy-to-digest foods and light soups that are kind to your system. This is also a great way to eliminate foods that have a negative effect on your digestion. Maintaining smaller, controlled portions is gentler on the digestive tract and has been a topic of conversation linked to longevity through the years. Chew your food as if you are digesting it in your mouth. This technique is great for smoothies and juices, too. Get the maximum nutrition from all the delicious, healthy foods you are eating!

BE FIT;
DON'T QUIT!

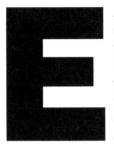xercise is the third pillar of a healthy lifestyle and the ultimate way to age with power. Nir Barzilai, M.D., director of the Institute for Aging Research at the Albert Einstein College of Medicine, is a scientist I met recently who studies longevity. He feels that exercise is critical for us as we age because not only does it build physical strength—important for muscle mass, flexibility, balance, and bone health—it helps us manage and recover from emotional stress. Dealing with stress is critical. Stress affects physical health and can compromise the immune system. Our bodies and minds retain the memory of pushing through a challenging workout, says Dr. Barzilai, so that when more stress presents itself in our lives, we are better equipped to navigate our way through it.

Studies show that regular exercise can lift mood, encourage better quality of sleep, boost immunity, improve cardiovascular health and brain function, and reduce the risk of chronic disease. It's great for your skin. It's energizing. It even perks up sex drive.

A flexible, strong body is youthful, and the way you move defines the perception of your age. I believe that a well-toned body and face are better than plastic surgery any day.

WORKING OUT SHOULD BE AS ROUTINE AS BRUSHING YOUR TEETH. ONCE YOU START EXERCISING EVERY DAY, IT BECOMES SECOND NATURE.

Working out should be as routine as brushing your teeth. Once you start exercising every day, it becomes second nature. You should change it up, but be consistent. During the week, I start my day early at six-thirty A.M. I am at work, and I have quiet time for design and new ideas. I pick four-thirty P.M. weekdays as my time to work out. I give my mind a rest and I enter a new zone. Some days I look forward to it and some days I don't, but I know one thing for sure is that I need to work out for balance and as a stress reliever, so I make it happen.

BE FIT; DON'T QUIT!

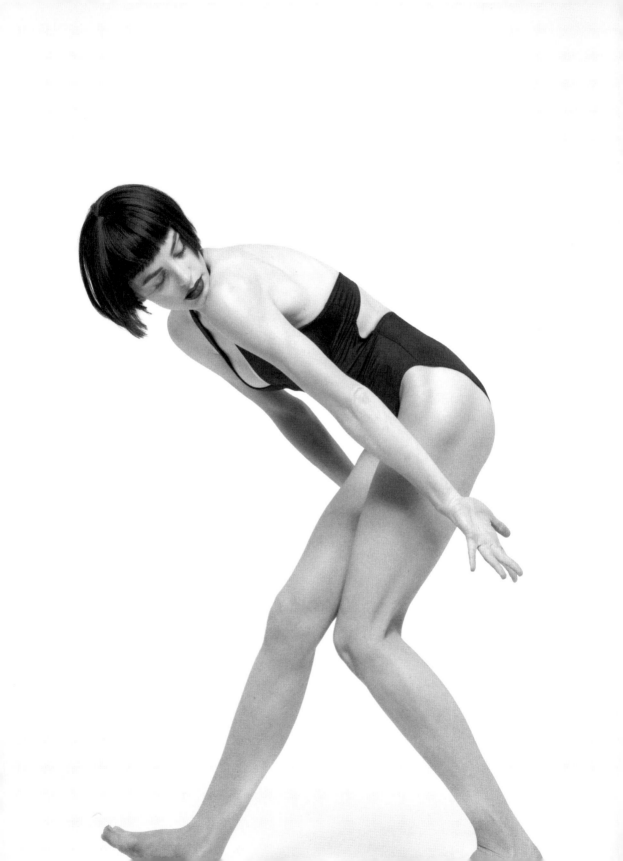

Exercise has always been important in my life. Before working out was mainstream, dancing was the universal activity. I think I danced daily, nonstop, until 1980! Back then, even sweaty gyms for men with weights were few and far between. Jane Fonda gave women a visual for what working out should look like. As we locked in our VHS cassettes, I memorized all of the routines and loved every video.

I love trying different types of exercise to see what they do for my body and overall well-being. Over the years, I have tried practically everything, from Gyrokinesis, tai chi, and circuit training with the famous Romanian trainer Radu to running, basketball (I can shoot thirty hoops in a row), yoga, and Maison Munz. I love to sweat. I love the feel of a workout burn. I love a toned body.

In the 1990s, I ventured over to a gym that claimed to be the headquarters of the authentic Pilates technique. It was a gymnastic area cohabited by the students of Joseph Pilates. Romana Kryzanowska was his original protégée, and with her group of hard-core ballet mistresses she taught the precision movements with strict Pilates accuracy.

I remember seeing gorgeous women of all ages into their sixties looking elegant and youthful with lithe dancers' bodies, and thinking, *Could that ever be me?* While I am hardly the ultimate shining example of the Joe Pilates technique (even though I try to be), I am ever grateful for the ten years I spent learning from the best. The principles of Pilates have evolved to become incorporated into almost every workout discipline we know today.

In 2006, when Physique 57—a new gym featuring a unique barre series—opened a few doors away from my office, I had no idea what it was, but I signed up for five classes. More than a decade later, I am still benefiting from the precise movements that rely on your own weight as resistance and exhaust each muscle group to literally shape the body. It's tough and transformative, physically and mentally.

As a result of trying new methodologies, seeking out new instructors, and taking the time to figure out what I like, I have learned to design the body I want.

BEFORE WORKING OUT WAS MAINSTREAM, DANCING WAS THE UNIVERSAL ACTIVITY.

I THINK I DANCED DAILY, NONSTOP, UNTIL 1980!

What I have discovered is this: fitness is a lifestyle.

No matter your budget or schedule or age, you can and should do some kind of physical activity every day. A great benefit of exercise is the power of mind over body when you push yourself beyond what you did the day before and reach a new personal goal. This translates easily into other goals you have in your life.

For those of you without a gym available, find a staircase. You can climb the stairs as many times as it takes to get your heart pumping, and increase the number of flights a little bit each week. You can start with one step at a time. The bottom line is you will come away with a workout.

Movement is important for everything in our lives. Making it a part of my life has been key to how I feel about my body and my self-esteem. There is something to be said for achieving what seemed impossible physically to inform you about what you can make possible in other parts of your life. NK

MY BODY IS MY HOME. BE FIT.

IF YOU CAN PUSH PAST THE CHALLENGES IN A WORKOUT, YOU MOST LIKELY CAN PUSH THROUGH THE CHALLENGES IN LIFE.

IF YOU TEST YOUR ABILITY TO GO FURTHER THAN YOU THINK YOU ARE CAPABLE OF GOING AND YOU SUCCEED, THEN YOU KNOW YOU CAN DO MORE.

ONCE YOU SURPASS OLD LIMITATIONS, YOU HAVE GIVEN YOURSELF PERMISSION TO **DREAM BIG DREAMS.**

IMAGINE THE STRENGTH, ENDURANCE, AND BODY YOU WANT.

THEN YOUR MIND AND BODY WILL CONNECT TO ACHIEVE THE RESULTS. YOUR BODY CAN DO SO MUCH MORE THAN YOU THINK IT CAN; YOU JUST HAVE TO TRAIN IT. THE RESULT OF ROUTINE EXERCISE IS THAT BY INCREASING THE CHALLENGES YOU ACHIEVE NEW GOALS.

AS THE OWNER OF A COMPANY, I SEE THAT THE PRODUCTIVITY OF STAFF MEMBERS WHO WORK OUT IS CLEARLY MUCH GREATER THAN THOSE WHO DO NOT. I OFFER TO HELP FINANCE MY TEAM'S FITNESS REGIMES IF THEY SHOW ME THEY EXERCISE TWELVE TIMES OR MORE EACH MONTH.

PICK A GYM OR WORKOUT NEAR YOU.

THE KEY IS CONVENIENCE—THEN YOU CAN BE CONSISTENT. THIS IS THE FIRST STEP TO SUCCESS.

BE FIT; DON'T QUIT!

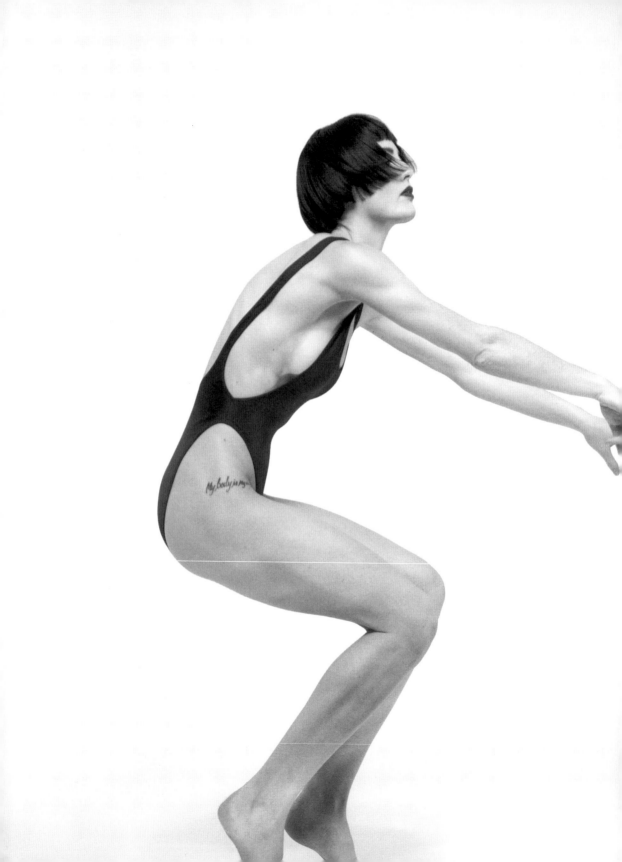

YOU CAN DESIGN THE BODY YOU WANT BY DOING SIMPLE EXERCISES.

EVERY TIME I WORK OUT, MY MOTIVATION IS TO HAVE THE TYPE OF BODY I WANT TO HAVE.

STRENGTHEN YOUR CORE;
IT CREATES THE BEST POSTURE.

DO PUSH-UPS AND PLANKS FOR PERKY
BREASTS AND TIGHT ABS.

DO LUNGES FOR TONED LEGS.

DO SQUATS FOR A SCULPTED BUTT.

USE WEIGHTS FOR CHISELED ARMS.

DO SCISSORS WITH EXTENDED STRAIGHT
LEGS FOR LONG, LEAN LEGS AND TIGHT ABS.

SQUEEZE A BALL BETWEEN YOUR LEGS
FOR FIRM INNER THIGHS AND AS A GREAT
KEGEL EXERCISE.

POSTURE...

...IS A CHALLENGE OF OUR TECHNOLOGY-DRIVEN LIVES. WHEN WE CURVE OVER AND LOOK DOWN INTO OUR DEVICES, OUR POSTURE SUFFERS.

TRY THIS:

EACH TIME YOU CHECK A TEXT OR PERSONAL MESSAGE OR MAKE A PHONE CALL, GET UP AND WALK AROUND, AND KEEP YOUR CHIN PARALLEL TO THE GROUND.

KEEP MOVING.

BLOOD FLOW TO THE BRAIN AND
BODY KEEPS EVERYTHING IN
GOOD WORKING ORDER. IF YOU
SIT ALL DAY, YOU NEED TO
GET UP AND MOVE AROUND. TAKE
THE STAIRS WHEN YOU HAVE
THE CHOICE. WHEN YOU ARE ON
A PLANE, GET UP AND MOVE.

MUSCLE MEMORY IS REAL.

IF YOU STOP EXERCISING AND
THEN START AGAIN, WITHIN A
PERIOD OF TIME YOUR BODY WILL
RETURN TO WHERE IT WAS BEFORE
STOPPING. I FIND THE LONGER
YOU ARE AWAY, THE LONGER IT
TAKES YOUR BODY TO RESPOND.
SO, WORD TO THE WISE . . .

GET BACK AS SOON AS YOU CAN.

RESPECT!

**YOUR BODY IMAGE
SAYS A LOT ABOUT YOUR
CONFIDENCE AND
SELF-ESTEEM. DURING
THE TIMES YOU ARE
THINKING OF SKIPPING
A WORKOUT, DON'T
GIVE UP OR GIVE IN TO
A WEAK MOMENT.**

DON'T CHEAT YOURSELF.

CHEATING EQUATES TO DISRESPECT.

IF YOU HAVE RESPECT FOR YOURSELF,

EVERYONE ELSE WILL, TOO.

BE FIT; DON'T QUIT!

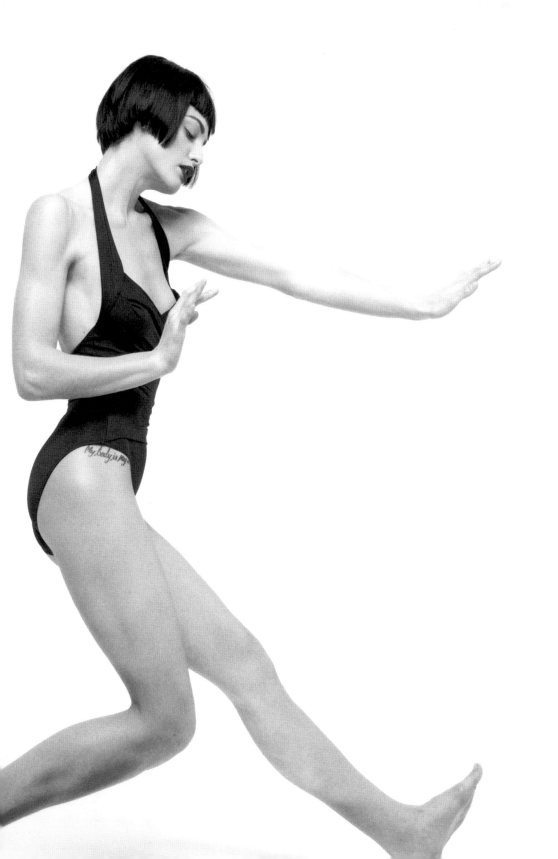

THE BASICS

I THINK OF EXERCISES IN TERMS OF THE MUSCLE GROUPS AND THE SECTION OF THE BODY I AM WORKING: ARMS, LEGS, CORE, THIGHS, AND BUTT. FOR A ONE-HOUR ROUTINE, I SPEND FIFTEEN MINUTES SHAPING EACH, ALWAYS ENGAGING MY ABS.

SIMPLE, TIMELESS TECHNIQUES ALWAYS WORK. AS YOU PROGRESS, YOU CAN COMBINE AND INVENT MORE CHALLENG-ING VERSIONS OF THE MOVES IN THIS SECTION. EVEN IF YOU STAY WITH THE CLASSIC, PROVEN MOVE-MENTS, JUST BY INCREAS-ING THE NUMBER OF REPS, OR BY ADDING ARM AND LEG WEIGHTS, YOU WILL INCREASE YOUR WORK-OUT'S INTENSITY.

GOOD FORM

The best workout is when your entire body is practicing perfect form head-to-toe to prevent injuries. **Thanks to Joseph Pilates, we understand that the core is the powerhouse of the body, from where all energy should emerge in order to perform a movement properly.** The alignment of all extensions comes from pushing energy out of the body through either the legs and feet or the arms and hands. Lift up through the ribs and engage the torso, pushing down through the hips and legs. Remember to keep the neck aligned straight through the spine to the top of the head. Reach up through the neck, as this is what creates elegant form. The pain you may feel after a full-body workout should be the burn and the building of muscle and tone, not an aching lower back from improper technique. **Good form is what creates the change.** All the move-ments I describe here are low-impact. By following correct form, you will strengthen your body and become less prone to injuries. Never push through pain. However, always consider pushing through the burn.

STRETCH

Stretch throughout the day and definitely after all workouts. The more time I spend stretching, the better I feel. Regular stretching increases circulation and keeps muscles lean, long, and flexible. For me, it is also a way to destress. **Breathing with the stretch is the secret. When you breathe and stretch, it is an active meditation.** Stretching increases flexibility, which is important for agility and positive body language. It improves balance and range of motion, which helps prevent injury. It's best to do when the body is warm and you are breathing with each movement. **You can increase your flexibility just by being able to touch your toes.** Try this tip below with soft knees, and with practice, soon you will be doing it with straight legs:

• Breathe in; lift up out of your torso, raising your arms and reaching for the sky.

• Stretch the space between your pelvis and rib cage to reach up and slowly reach over to touch your toes as you exhale one long, strong breath.

Listen to your body. If you need to stretch, take the time. It's like a big, head-to-toe yawn.

BREATHE

Breathe through every exercise to achieve your best form and to gain the maximum productivity in order to take you beyond your expectations. Bringing fresh oxygen into the body with controlled inhalations, while exhaling carbon dioxide, promotes the best results. It's simple: If you try working out and you are not breathing, the exercise will be much harder. There are many health benefits associated with mindful breathwork. It has been shown to help reduce insomnia, anxiety, stress, and ADD, to increase alertness, and to boost the immune system. I initially learned how to breathe while I exercise through practicing Pilates. **Every type of movement is performed better when the rhythm of your breath matches the rhythm of the exercise.** In certain classes, the actual sound of inhaling and exhaling helps remind us how important breathing is for all exercise and how much further we go in our practice with breath support. The yogic breath is in through the nose and out through the nose, creating an ocean wave sound. Pilates is in through the nose and out through the mouth, with purpose. Gyrokinesis teaches us to breathe in through the nose and blow out through the mouth, producing a rhythmic sound. Every motion is in sync with the breath.

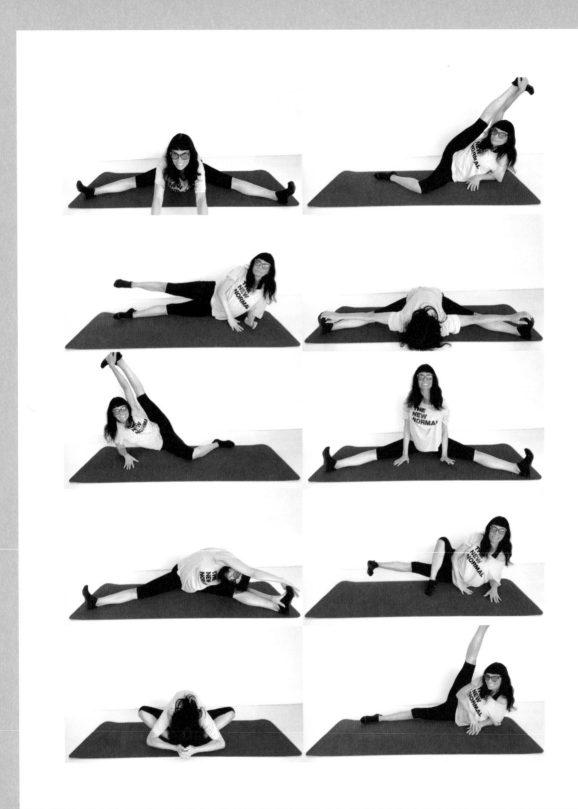

MAKE EXERCISE FIT YOUR HABITS

FOR THOSE OF YOU WHO MISS YOUR WORKOUT OR PREFER TO EXERCISE ALONE, FOLLOWING A LIVE-STREAM CLASS IS A GREAT OPTION. IF I MISS A CLASS AND AM AT HOME, OR AM TRAVELING AND IN A HOTEL ROOM, I STILL MAKE IT FIT.

I am a multitasker and find it impossible to watch a video, TV show, or movie without feeling like I am accomplishing something. Therefore, I keep a collection of stretchy looped resistance bands nearby, which I use for an hour-long series of ab, arm, butt, and thigh exercises while I watch. I time the exercise series to the length of the show, so by the time it is finished, so am I. Sometimes I use two bands—one for arms and upper body and another for thighs and legs. Props like bands are great because they support the fact that you are truly working out. They are also the easiest, most travel-friendly prop. I take mine everywhere.

HERE ARE A FEW BASIC ROUTINES ANYONE CAN FOLLOW.

NORMA'S ROUTINE

A SIMPLE PLAN FOR BEGINNERS

This is an extremely simple routine and good for all ages. If you have an injury, have never worked out in your life, or are older and feeling stiffness and discomfort, this might get you up and moving. Remember, everyone started out as a beginner. The more consistent you are and the more you do, the better you get at it. Your body has muscle memory, so you will always be ahead of where you started. Resistance bands are incredible for creating real results you can see. I use looped bands, though you can also knot straight bands to create a taut, circular shape. They are available in different thicknesses—the thicker the band, the higher the resistance. Start light and as you progress, increase the resistance. Add reps in increments of twenty or fifty for an increased challenge and as you gain strength.

1 ARMS

EXERCISE 1

Sit cross-legged, leaning slightly forward with shoulders back and a flat back. Or stand with feet hip-distance apart and knees slightly bent.

Extend your arms straight behind you and place both hands inside the circular band, pushing outward so the rubber is taut.

With straight arms, do little lifts upward—small pulses—in a rhythmic count.

Start with twenty pulses. For more of a challenge, add more reps.

EXERCISE 2

Sitting or standing, place both hands inside the band and raise your arms straight overhead, with shoulders down.

Keeping the band taut, fold your forearms down, back behind your head, so your hands touch your shoulders and your elbows are facing up to the ceiling (the band will be extended across the back of your neck). Lift your arms up to the ceiling, continuing to press out on the band to maintain tension. Briefly pause at the top, and repeat the motion. Start with twenty reps. This is a great extension for the triceps and shoulders.

EXERCISE 3

Stand with both arms straight overhead, hands inside the band.

As you bend to the left, arching the right side of your body to curve toward the left, keep your right arm straight overhead while your left arm pulls the taut band down toward the left side, with elbow bent.

Do a pulsing count of twenty repetitions, creating a bicep curl, and then repeat on the opposite side.

2 ABS

EXERCISE 1

Sit on the floor, leaning comfortably back on your forearms, with elbows directly under shoulders, curved back, and shoulders pressed down.

Place the band around your feet, separating your feet to create tension, and lift both legs off the ground.

With legs raised, abs engaged, and arms planted firmly on the ground, simulate running in place: extending one flexed foot out forward, with control, while the opposite knee bends in toward the chest, for fifty repetitions.

Feel free to either speed it up or slow it down; just keep the rhythm consistent.

EXERCISE 2

Lie on your back with straight legs stretched up to the ceiling, band around arches of the feet, with your legs separated hip-distance apart to create tension, and feet flexed.

Slowly pulse your legs outward, creating more tension with the band. Keep your hips anchored to the ground, legs straight, abs engaged, and shoot energy out through the heels, for fifty reps.

This seems easy until you get to the fifteenth rep! This movement works your abs, thighs, and butt, and the more you do, the more you'll feel it's working.

EXERCISE 3

Sitting on the floor, place the band around the arches of both feet and pull the band up between your legs with both hands, creating a diamond shape with your legs. Anchor your heels into the ground and flex both feet.

Engaging your abs, scoop back as far as you can go, with straight arms pulling the band taut. Slowly roll up, halfway, and then roll back down, holding the pose.

Do that twenty times and, let me tell ya, you'll feel it.

3 THIGHS

EXERCISE 1

Stand with the band around both ankles and your feet slightly turned out, holding on to a barre or the wall, if desired.

With one foot planted firmly on the floor, push out to the side with the other, and with pointed toes, trace a small circle. After twenty circles counterclockwise, with the same foot, reverse direction.

Repeat with the opposite leg.

EXERCISE 2

Lie on your side with the band around both legs, placed above bended knees. With feet together, slowly open and close your knees, creating a diamond shape, with a slight pulse each time you open.

After twenty reps, switch sides.

EXERCISE 3

Lying back, prop your upper body on your elbows, forearms facing forward. Place the band around your ankles; legs are straight and hip-distance apart.

With one foot pressing firmly into the floor, and abs engaged, lift the opposite foot (either pointed or flexed) for twenty small pulses upward. Switch feet. This sounds so simple, but the resistance the band creates is really major. It's great for the thighs, but you're also lifting with the abs.

EXERCISE 4

Place the band around your ankles. Lie on your stomach and place your hands under your forehead.

With straight legs and pointed toes, one leg remains flat with the foot pressing into the ground, while the other lifts as high as it can, in a pulsing movement, for twenty counts.

Repeat with the opposite leg.

4 BUTT

EXERCISE 1

On all fours with flat back, knees hip-distance apart, place the band around both legs, above the knees.

With your right knee anchored to floor, lift your left knee, rotating the leg out to the left side. Pause, and release. Repeat for twenty reps, and then switch legs.

EXERCISE 2

Place the band above your right knee and the arch of your right foot. On hands and knees with a flat back, extend your right foot toward the ceiling in small, controlled pulses, for twenty counts.

Switch legs.

EXERCISE 3

Standing, place the band above your knees and sink into a traditional squat.

Separating your knees to create tension with the band, lower farther into a seated squat. Repeat, lowering and lifting with a slight pulse, for twenty counts.

THE CLASSIC 5

For each movement, increase repetitions over time.

1 CRUNCHES	2 LUNGES	3 SQUATS	4 PUSH-UPS	5 PLANKS
START WITH 50 REPS	START WITH 30 REPS EACH LEG	START WITH 30 REPS	START WITH 30 REPS	START WITH 20 SECONDS

THE POSTURE SERIES

EXERCISE 1

This is my version of "swimming," adapted from the classical Pilates technique.

Lie facedown on a mat.

Ground hipbones, pelvis, and lower abs to the floor.

Reach straight arms out front with extended fingers, and extend straight legs back with pointed toes.

Extend your neck and lift your head, eyes facing forward. Lift your shoulders, arms, and legs, hip-distance apart. With lifted chest and energy shooting out in opposite directions, lower and lift alternate arm with alternate leg. Keep switching for twenty counts, for a fluid, kicking motion that mimics swimming.

EXERCISE 2

This is great for the back muscles.

Props: small (playground-size) exercise ball and 2-pound weights.

Sit on the floor with the ball positioned behind your back.

Take one weight in each hand and stretch back, arching over the ball, so your head is facing back and your arms are outstretched. Legs can be extended, or knees can be bent, with feet on the floor, hip-distance apart.

Spread your arms over the ball like wings, so the weights are now resting on the floor, palms down.

With your chest open, lift the weights with slightly bent elbows to chest height, rhythmically pulsing in counts of four, twenty times.

EXERCISE 3 Shoulder Blade Kiss

Seated or standing, extend straight arms and clasp your hands behind your back.

As your chest opens, attempt to touch your shoulder blades together.

With chin lifted, pulse straight arms with clasped hands upward twenty times in slow, intentional lifts.

You should be exhausted now. If you do these regularly, you'll begin to see good things happen. They really do work.

AGE WITH POWER

THE DECADES

IF YOU FELT YOU WOULD GET BETTER WITH AGE,
HOW WOULD YOU LIVE YOUR LIFE?

EVERY DECADE COMES WITH A DIFFERENT SET OF CHALLENGES AND OPPORTUNITIES.

OUR FIRST HORMONAL BLAST BEGINS WHEN WE ENTER PUBERTY, AND THESE UPS AND DOWNS STAY WITH US UNTIL WE EXIT MENOPAUSE. THIS IS A RIDE NO ONE TELLS US ABOUT, AND WE GO THROUGH IT LIKE THE INCREDIBLY POWERFUL BEINGS WE ARE.

MANEUVERING SUCCESSFULLY THROUGH LIFE'S PASSAGES INCLUDES THESE PHYSICAL AND SPIRITUAL TRANSITIONS. REINVENTING OURSELVES ALONG THE WAY, FEELING GOOD ABOUT OURSELVES AND OUR ABILITY TO BE RELEVANT, IS THE GOAL.

THIS IS MY DECADE-BY-DECADE GUIDE TO MOVING THROUGH LIFE WITH PURPOSE, AND THE STORIES OF HOW I NAVIGATED KEY MOMENTS OF MY OWN, FROM THE FAILURES AND INSTANCES OF UNCERTAINTY TO THE TRIUMPHS.

EVERYONE HAS A DIFFERENT PATH AND PLAN. REACHING YOUR POTENTIAL DOESN'T HAVE A DATE. AGING WITH POWER IS HOW YOU GET THERE.

TEENs
SURPRISE!
PIMPLES, PERIODS, AND PUBERTY

20s
YOU'RE NOT A KID ANYMORE
PRETENDING UNTIL WE FIGURE IT OUT

30s
WHOOPS, WHAT JUST HAPPENED?
LIFE'S BIG CHALLENGES GET REAL

40s
I KNOW WHO I AM, AND I AM MAKING IT HAPPEN
HELLO, HORMONES, DON'T MESS WITH ME NOW

50s
OHHHH BOY, REINVENTION!
BIG CHANGES BEGIN—FINALLY, MAYBE LONG OVERDUE

60s
UNFILTERED, UNEDITED
IT'S ME, IT'S ME, IT'S ME AT LAST!

70s
IF YOU ONLY KNEW
LIVE YOUR PURPOSE

80s, 90s ...100
KEEP DANCING!

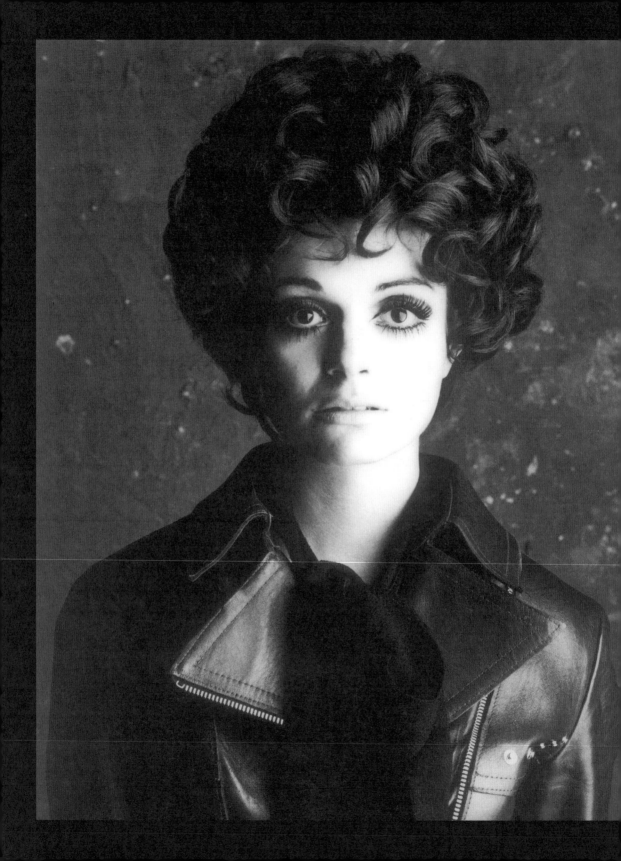

TEENs

THIS IS WHEN THE EMOTIONAL AND PHYSICAL CRASH COURSE INTO WOMANHOOD, AND SELFHOOD, BEGINS.

The hormonal roller coaster women experience during their lifetime spans from puberty to menopause. We have become more open and engaged in conversations about menopause, but puberty is still quietly handled in an assortment of random discussions.

My memories of puberty are very clear because it was so abrupt. My tomboy childhood was active, and my angular body fit the fence-climbing, swimming, jumping, physical life of a kid.

While riding my brother's bike down a hill one afternoon when I was twelve years old, I skidded sideways into a tree and landed on the bar across the boys' bike. There was blood on my white shorts. I went up to our apartment to show my mother and tell her I probably had internal bleeding from my accident.

AGE EIGHTEEN. IT ONLY TOOK A WIG, FALSE EYELASHES, PANCAKE MAKEUP, AND AN HOUR AND A HALF TO GET THIS LOOK!

143

She didn't sit me down to tell me this was the beginning of my rite of passage into womanhood and that I would have the ability to bear children and call upon the special traits women have for nurturing and motherhood. What she did do was hand me a Kotex pad (an enormous-size one that fit her adult body perfectly, but was certainly not going to be tucked away for convenience on my much smaller frame). She instructed that I would use these monthly and showed me where they were stored in the cabinet for future use. Wow. Thankfully, Tampax came along, and today there are many easy-to-use choices that allow women to be as active as we want to be during our period.

The next thing I noticed was that my body was changing, with the appearance of breasts, rounded hips, a sensitivity to touch, and a new silhouette in clothing. The boys and men in my world were looking at me in a different way, and I was aware of the fact that they were looking at my body. Adjusting to this was a confused effort on my part because I wasn't clear about the messages, especially since I was not completely comfortable in my own skin.

Oh yes, skin. Pimples ... where did these come from? I didn't have a lot, but I swear it seemed I always had a blemish on my face. I was self-conscious about my body, my blemishes, my nose, which was growing out of control, and this newfound maturity I was pretending to be able to handle.

I remember my first kiss around this time, as well. A sensation I could not imagine before and quite frankly didn't truly understand. Feeling a boy's hand on my body was so confusing because I felt an invasion of my private space. However, there was another part of me that thought, *He is attracted to me*, and I could sense the excitement and appreciation this boy appeared to have for this experience, which made me feel special.

Women have a compelling desire to be loved. In my fifty-plus years as an adult around women, I have been witness to and have personally experienced this inclination that begins at puberty and follows us throughout our lives. Sometimes it even manifests itself in allowing ourselves to be objectified if we sense there is an opportunity for love and affection.

I will never forget the scene in the movie *Bridesmaids* when Kristen Wiig is in bed with Jon Hamm and he has clearly used the opportunity she presented to his own advantage. Even though she knew his interest in her was limited and on his terms, she believed that over time she would win him over. Well, of course not! As I looked at that scene, I realized that I have foolishly participated in my own version of that very same scenario. And I wondered if this isn't a super-common experience among women of all ages in their steadfast desire to be loved.

I work with women and have appointments with women throughout the day, every day, and my friends are women. So this observation needed a survey, and yes, unanimously, every women I asked acknowledged that she, too, had done the same thing in some form, secretly believing that with perseverance she would win over the love interest. And almost without exception we all failed. The result usually ended in humiliation, embarrassment, and pain, and yet many repeated the behavior again and again.

FEELING BEAUTIFUL IS INCREDIBLY IMPORTANT FOR WOMEN, AND EARLY ON, AS INSECURE TEENAGERS, WE INEVITABLY BECOME CONVINCED THAT IT IS DEFINED BY EVERYTHING THAT EVERYONE ELSE IS AND WE ARE NOT.

This and other early objectification experiences lead to self-esteem issues. There is added confusion with the first signs of competitive friendships and mean-girl manifestations, many times related to romantic relationships.

Then we add in the pretty factor. Feeling beautiful is incredibly important for women, and early on, as insecure teenagers, we inevitably become convinced that it is defined by everything that everyone else is and we are not. The beauty and fashion industries have traditionally set the standard for what beauty looks like (thank goodness this is changing), and the standard is, and has been, unrealistic.

Unfortunately, social media is now replacing magazines in presenting limited, impractical notions of beauty by adding filters not unlike the airbrushing traditionally used in advertisements and editorials to promote flawless aspirational ideals. The residual effects can be particularly wounding to young viewers who do not yet realize that being an original beauty—an authentic woman with a brain and a soul and a look all her own—cannot be duplicated and should be celebrated with confidence.

The experience of puberty is the first passage in a woman's life that teaches us that self-love is how we ride the roller coaster through the highs and lows and come out all the better for it. Recognizing the importance of self-respect, cultivating the power of a confident mind and developing a strong body, and the ability to achieve self-love require tools.

A healthy lifestyle, built around the Three Pillars of sleep, diet, and exercise, is how you learn to own your mind-body power. This is the foundation that will help develop the positive identity that will define you. You will attract the people you deserve and the opportunities you deserve. These are tools for life, and the earlier you start using them, the more empowered you will be throughout everything that comes at you.

Diet can affect everything from your mood and your behavior to how you look. Many times our relationship with food becomes complicated and we are influenced by trendy diets or unhealthy eating habits. It's possible to achieve a healthy body that is powerful and at the proportionate weight for your height and bone mass without using scales or measurements.

How much you eat and the quality of what you eat are one part of the fit-body factor. Food with nutrition is important for not just overall health but how you look and how you feel mentally. I consider food that is junk as something that makes me look like junk, feel like junk, and think like junk. It's easy to slip when you are in a hurry or feeling stressed, but by choosing good food, you are reversing the mind and body's perception of how you feel and who you are. In the Food chapter of this book, there are some guidelines, but as a teen, put colorful plant-based snacks between you and sugar, dairy, and caffeine. Lots of water and low-sugar smoothies (meaning use berries instead of high-sugar fruits) with nutritional green powders for an extra vitamin boost are great for nutrition and energy. Needless to say, fried foods and processed snacks bloat your body, slow down your energy, dampen your outlook, and are absolutely not great for your complexion. Shiny hair, glowing skin, and sparkly eyes all are achieved through the food you eat, not the beauty department.

> **RECOGNIZING THE IMPORTANCE OF SELF-RESPECT, CULTIVATING THE POWER OF A CONFIDENT MIND AND A STRONG BODY, AND DEVELOPING THE ABILITY TO ACHIEVE SELF-LOVE REQUIRE TOOLS.**

Exercise not only gives you a strong body, but also teaches you that things you never thought you could do can be achieved with practice and effort, and this translates to life goals and aspirations.

There is no drug as positive for building confidence as the energy, endorphins, and feeling you have after a workout—and then, how you look as a result. Your body-positive image comes to life. I would take working out over drugs and alcohol any day. Drugs and alcohol are temporary highs that dull the senses. Exercise positively enhances the senses and self-esteem does not come in a bottle.

There are so many choices for exercise. Try things more than once, say five times, and decide what suits you. I always refer to the staircase as the most affordable gym. You can go up and down stairs as many times as you like and keep aiming for more. You can do it fast—two steps, three steps at a time—to get the blood flowing, deliver oxygen to cells, and work up a sweat. This releases toxins and all of the emotional stuff you want to clean out of your mind. It also opens pores, which can help improve skin.

Sleep helps restore every cell in your body from the emotional and physical wear and tear each day imposes. Not only will you think more clearly and feel better about yourself when you are well-rested, you will look better, too.

Meditation is like a clean sweep for any stress that impacts the day, helping you to remain calm, balanced, and in control of how you feel. You can do it anywhere, anytime, and the more you do it, the better you will be at it. The ability to center yourself is incredibly powerful. Meditation and breathwork both support sleep, and all three support you through every tough situation that comes your way. You will find that the ability to be kind comes so easily when you are practicing each daily.

This is also the best time to start thinking about your purpose in this lifetime and developing big, wonderful dreams that inspire hope and a positive outlook. Kindness is a way to discover your purpose and how you will serve for the good and understand and create your relevance in the world.

What you learn now you will carry with you for the rest of your life. The habits you form—taking care of your body and mind—will shape how you evolve and handle situations. This is the time to start making good habits your habits. **NK**

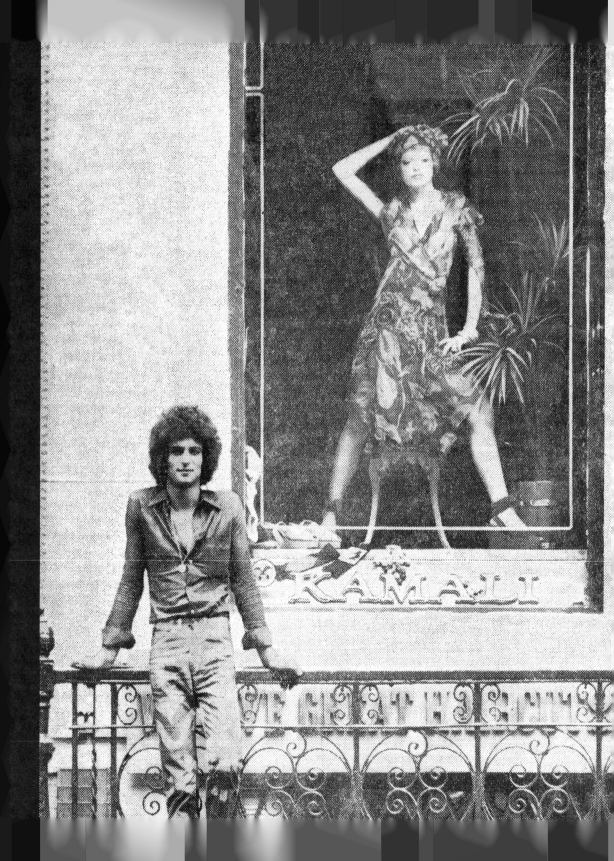

20s

TURNING TWENTY IS THE REALIZATION THAT YOU ARE NOT A TEEN ANYMORE AND YOU WILL HAVE TO START TAKING ON ADULT RESPONSIBILITIES.

When I turned eighteen, my mother said, "Happy birthday—it's all downhill from here!" I had tears in my eyes because I really believed she might be right. I was no longer a kid, and that meant I would get old like everyone over nineteen. Nonetheless, I decided to move forward with an optimistic attitude as I expanded my life experience. Age was not going to deter me because I was a Boomer—we were changing everything in every way. We were different, and weren't we going to live forever?

My training from the start was to be a painter. I won painting awards, grants, and scholarships, but my mother was nervous for my financial security if I followed that path. I also received a scholarship for fashion illustration from the Fashion Institute of

MANSOUR KAMALI, MY HUSBAND, IN FRONT OF OUR SHOP, WITH ME IN THE WINDOW.
WE WERE FEARLESS AND DETERMINED.

149

Technology. My mother convinced me to look at that as my security. I could always paint if I had a job.

After graduating from FIT, I was enthusiastic and ready to enter the job market. I prepared my fashion illustration portfolio with as much love and care and detail as I could to create something that would make a powerful impact during my job interviews.

My first interview was memorable but impossible to talk about until ten years ago.

From the time we are born, girls are judged by the way we look, and that will be the focus of much of the objectification we experience. Throughout my life I have withstood countless instances of objectification, and like every other woman, I learned to manage my life around those moments, determined to reach my goals.

For my first interview, not only did I prepare an impeccable portfolio, I meticulously planned my outfit, hair, makeup, shoes, everything. I remember what I wore as if it were yesterday: a little black dress with black pumps, my hair pulled back in a low ponytail, and minimal makeup—basically mascara and nude lips matching my skin tone. I was wearing the typical undergarments of the time: a garter belt, stockings, a cotton no-stretch bra, and panties of cotton, as well.

Off I went to the Garment District, and as I entered the building's lobby, with its marble floors and shiny elevator, my enormous portfolio started tearing streaks of runs in my stockings along my left leg. Horrified, I thought to myself, *I can't turn around; I need to just get into the interview and make it happen.* I was determined on the inside but quiet on the outside, shy.

I was escorted into an office, and there was a man sitting with his feet up on the desk, eating a tuna sandwich! He directed me to put my portfolio against the wall and step over to his desk. I followed his instructions, and as I stood in front of him, he told me to *turn around*. My mind went blank except for my mother's voice saying I'd better get a job because she was not going to support me much longer. He was the power in the room, so I turned around! I was so humiliated and embarrassed, I grabbed my portfolio and ran out of the office in tears. I told my mother I didn't get the job and quickly looked in the *New York Times* employment section for anything.

Every experience puts us on either a path we should be on, or one we should not. I didn't realize it at the moment, but the trauma of that event pushed me to pursue a new direction that led to my dreams.

At this time, in the early sixties, the airlines were the cool, futuristic jobs of the moment, like Apple later became for technology. There was a position available at Northwest Orient Airlines in Reservations. I had absolutely zero office skills. I did not type or have any idea what I was interviewing for, but I had worked since I was twelve (at my stepdad's candy store), and the idea of travel excited me, so I thought I would give it a try. I was really surprised when they actually hired me. I decided I was going to be the best I could be at this job, and my competitive spirit really went into full force when all of the folks on staff from Minneapolis (except for one other girl) were sure that New Yorkers wouldn't be able to work at their level! Well, not only did we learn how to use some of the first computers in the workplace, we were amazingly productive. I sat at my Univac terminal and worked my way to International Sales in the Tour department.

Above all else in the life of a woman in her twenties, exploration in order to find one's true self is the dominant theme. The more curiosity you have experiencing life and trying things you may not be able to do at other times, the better. This decade is when it should happen.

On a discounted twenty-nine-dollar round-trip ticket, I traveled every weekend to London, where a disruptive, amazing revolution was taking place that still reverberates today. There I was every weekend for four years, in the center of the universe of rebellion, creativity, and change! I felt so much excitement being in this hotbed of pop-cultural activity where new ideas about fashion, music, and film were exploding into daily life.

I would scour the vintage markets for one-of-a-kind finds and shop at Biba and Bus Stop for styles no one had ever seen before. The Biba aesthetic was about empire-waist minidresses and miniskirts, pants and vests paired with skimpy jackets. Hats were a must-have; floppy brims worn with aviator sunglasses were my favorite.

The really fun part about one's twenties is the discovery of personal style. You have the freedom to dress any way you like at this time, so experimenting is the way to do it. Who you are and how you express yourself will change a

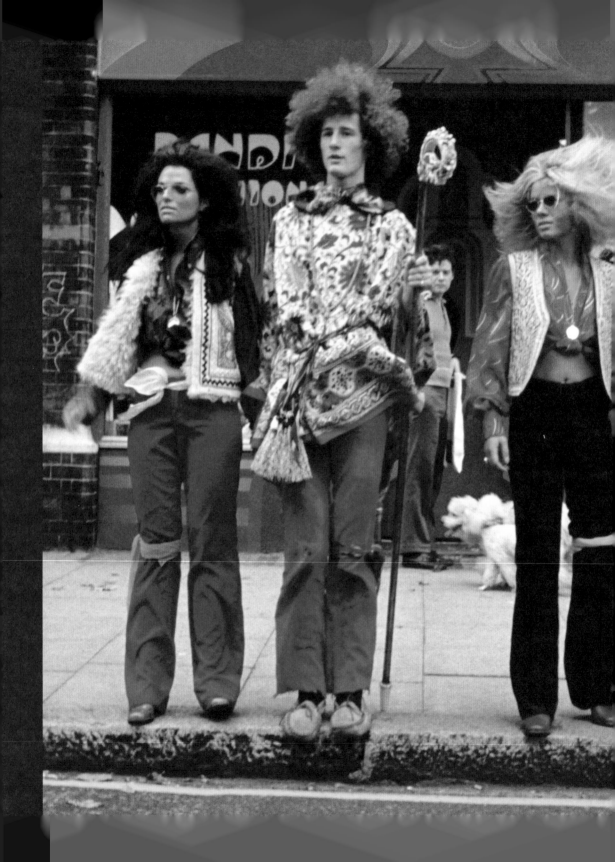

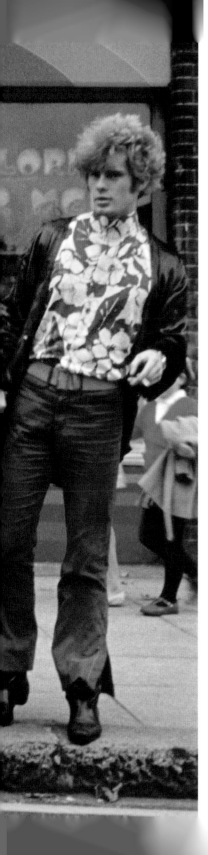

lot through this decade, and it should, because you are changing all the time.

The impact of this revolution on my imagination and the influence of what I could do became so clear! I decided that instead of being a painter, I now knew I wanted to design clothing. The matching-hat-and-bag *Mad Men* fashion of the early sixties that was so ubiquitous in New York was not my intuitive style, but innovation, invention, and design fit my intuitive nature.

In London, I found my voice. After bringing so many Biba and Bus Stop styles back for friends, I decided to open a store. I found a tiny, nine-by-twelve-foot basement space in a cluster of brownstones on East Fifty-Third Street for $285 a month. I hand-painted the floor and found a display case and snakeskin wallpaper at the Salvation Army. At the shop, called KAMALI, I sold pieces from London, and pretty soon I started designing my own styles. It was so much work, but I was in a dream.

At eighteen, I thought I knew everything. My twenties taught me how much I needed to learn but also fired the passion I had had for as long as I could remember to lead a creative life. I was in touch with who I was becoming.

I was extremely shy, and hidden behind the scenes designing I found a safe place. I believed in myself even though my lack of experience was glaring. In fact, I used it in my favor. I didn't let fear rule my decisions, and every time someone bought something, I was energized.

Celebrities like Diana Ross, Cher, Bianca Jagger, Diane Von Furstenberg, Donna Summer, and Raquel Welch found their way to me. My designs always considered how the clothes would look and feel in motion, so

WITH FRIENDS ON THE KING'S ROAD. LONDON IN THE SEVENTIES WAS A COSTUME PARTY!

they became the go-to for a good time. Both men and women discovered my underground store. Robert Plant shopped for full-sleeved shirts; I made feathered jackets in countless colors for Sly Stone. The New York Dolls were the city's it-group of the moment. They were the epitome of gender-fluid style, from their clothes to their makeup, nails, and accessories, and my shop was their closet! John Lennon would come in with Yoko. They were such a great couple and always had a witty exchange going. He was so funny and would do a dry commentary while he lounged on the banquettes as Yoko modeled each outfit.

Press in *Vogue* and *Harper's Bazaar* came early. The recognition gave me the encouragement to keep going even in the most difficult early years. I was so insecure, and was sure everyone would find out I really didn't know anything and that I was discovering it all along the way.

Inexperience really tested my abilities to be the boss as I hired people to help me make the clothing. I had not studied patternmaking or design, so I had to learn on the job. The people I hired were older, and, needless to say, they took advantage of my inexperience, telling me things were impossible to make, taking naps and breaks and generally bossing me around! This inspired me to make sure I learned every aspect of my world, from pattern-making and displays to sales, planning, purchasing—everything, so I could be the authority! I can proudly say my skills developed quite nicely, and I would still challenge any swimwear patternmaker in the world!

While I was designing and doing all of the production behind the scenes, my husband was beautiful and charming and selling the clothes. We grew and expanded a few times.

I met my husband at the first club in NYC that had a DJ instead of live music. We both knew the DJ, and he introduced us and suggested we enter the dance contest . . . Yes, dance contest! Well, we did, and we won five hundred dollars! He was alone in New York studying economics, his family all back in Iran; my mother was clearly not getting through menopause easily, and I needed to leave the house. I was nineteen, and girls just didn't move in back then; they got married. Okay, so he was

OKAY, SO HE WAS GOOD-LOOKING AND WE DANCED GREAT TOGETHER— IT WAS OBVIOUSLY DESTINY, RIGHT?

good-looking and we danced great together—it was obviously destiny, right?

The twenties are an intense time in the conventional life plan society has prescribed for women. We are expected to find a mate, get married, and be ready to have kids by thirty. It's a tremendous amount of pressure. The deadline is unrealistic and often makes for poor choices and long-term commitments involving relationships, children, and finances.

We all have our own timeline. The twenties are the moment to start to define your goals and how you want to see them materialize. Everything is ahead, and you are the author of your dream.

So much was happening in my life at this time. Aging didn't seem like something that would happen to me or my friends. I decided I would be young forever. Even though I knew this was not possible, I didn't let getting older enter my mind.

I ate bacon-blue-cheese burgers while smoking Salem cigarettes with my red-polished nails (fortunately, smoking for me only lasted a few years), topping it off with a piece of grape Bubblicious chewing gum for dessert. I danced all the time from sixteen years old on, and was always out and about. In the 1960s and '70s, dancing was our gym.

When I started designing (and was still working my day job at the airline—the early shift, from six A.M. to two P.M.), I didn't go dancing as often; there just wasn't time.

Health wasn't a priority for anyone my age, and the idea of a balanced lifestyle that considered diet, exercise, and sleep was not even thought about. What we did have in our favor was the fact that fast-food farming and pesticides weren't dominant and air pollution was so much less than it is today. We were lucky to have an environment that was safer. There were only three TV channels, and I remember listening to Martin Luther King Jr., JFK, and Gandhi influencing our spirit and inspiring the population. We were landing on the moon, and everything felt hopeful.

Drugs were everywhere, but I was not comfortable being out of control, especially not wanting to waste this incredible discovery of my ability to design clothing people were responding to so nicely. My goals were clear, and I couldn't let anything get in the way. NK

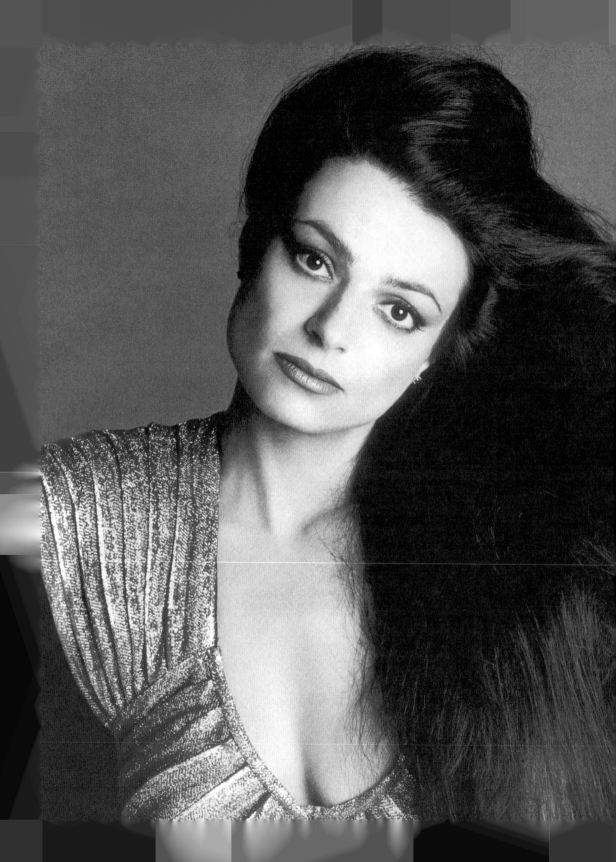

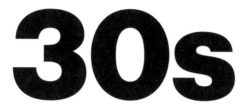

30s

TURNING THIRTY IS A BIG ONE.

THE FIRST GROWN-UP LIFE CHALLENGE USUALLY HITS AROUND THIS TIME. MINE WAS LEAVING MY HUSBAND, AND MY BUSINESS.

I t is very likely that a marriage between two nineteen-year-olds might have challenges. Ten years later we were divorced. I was twenty-nine, turning thirty. I was advised that if I ever left the company I could not take anything with me at all.

My husband was very social and went out every night. He was openly seeing other women, including a friend of mine and one of our salesgirls. We had taken two very different paths. He was a dominating presence, and feeling humiliated by his indiscretions was making it impossible for me to be with him as my husband or business partner.

It always takes a trigger to push you to the next place. Perhaps this is part of the Universe's plan for each of us. I was willing to tolerate a lot of the bullying if I could do what I loved. The concern I had constantly was having enough money to buy fabric. So seeing gifts of Rolex watches to the salesgirl was, needless to say, upsetting. Yes, I did fire her, but my husband rehired her. They lived a nightlife of parties and extravagance. He used the money we made for everything but company expenses. These were times when women believed men were better with money, so he controlled the money, and it was his way to control me.

I finally moved out to my own apartment, but with absolutely nothing, not even the dogs! (The first of many miniature dachshunds I've had through the years.) Still, it seemed impossible for me to walk away from the company I worked so hard to build. How could I leave everything behind, including my identity? The last straw was when the salesgirl came to the sample room to tell me she wanted me to make her customized designs and described in detail what they should look like. When she left the room, the ceiling over my cutting table literally fell! I thought to myself, *If there was a fortune cookie I were to read now, it would say, "When the ceiling falls on your head, time to leave!!"* So I left—and, oh, did I mention, I only had ninety-eight dollars to my name?

I had to leave all of my special fabrics, trims, patterns, and inspirations and start from scratch. But I was bringing with me ten years of experience and my point of view.

I had a mattress but no curtains, no furniture—nothing but my clothing. I did not have a plan. I was scared and unprepared, but at the same time I felt relief. My soul and my self-esteem were intact.

Coincidentally, at this time I had a rare meeting scheduled with an editor from the *Los Angeles Times*. I kept the appointment. She asked me if I was okay, because my face was swollen from crying and I was shaking. I explained I was no longer at KAMALI. For the first time in my life I talked about myself. When I told her my story, she offered help! I'd never thought of asking anyone for help, and I'd never thought anyone would offer it. Well, she did! Her husband happened to work in the

I HAD A MATTRESS BUT NO CURTAINS, NO FURNITURE— NOTHING BUT MY CLOTHING. I DID NOT HAVE A PLAN. I WAS SCARED AND UNPREPARED, BUT AT THE SAME TIME I FELT RELIEF. MY SOUL AND MY SELF-ESTEEM WERE INTACT.

garment industry, and he had a lot of connections. She took charge and said, "He can get you sewing machines!" Wow! I received similar offers of help from so many other people in and outside of the industry, and I was overwhelmed with appreciation.

OMO NORMA KAMALI was my new logo. It stood for ON MY OWN.

I would now be responsible for every aspect of the company, from design to running the business. The reason I didn't fear this role was that my desire to live a creative life without limits meant absolute freedom if I could stay in business and responsibly pay the bills. This was my life goal, and I would make all of my decisions based on that concept.

I paid back everyone who had lent me money, and when I was short of cash I would send a note apologizing and then follow up shortly with a payment plan. The business was doing well and there was so much press about me, a fashion designer going out on her own, a woman OMO in 1976! This seemed to be big news.

The seventies were an interesting time for feminism. The movement was starting to build with talk of women's opportunities and rights. The funny thing was, I was so focused on survival I literally had no connection to the movement and didn't really know what was going on. I never felt angry about the uneven gender privilege or even thought about it; however, I was living it like so many other women. Not realizing I was a feminist, I had simply decided that I needed to do what I wanted, not as a woman, but as a person with a dream.

The incredible outcome of my ON MY OWN statement was that so many women were inspired and moved to do something for themselves. I received letters and calls and ON MY OWN became a mantra for many other women.

The salesgirl and other painful experiences during my marriage affected my self-esteem and at times broke my heart. What I know now is that each situation forced me to move forward personally to get me where I was meant to go. I learned how important friction is in a person's life in order to motivate change.

There is no question my dignity was at stake. If I had stayed, my soul would have been lost, and I can't imagine I would have survived the experience. Leaving allowed my personal growth to continue.

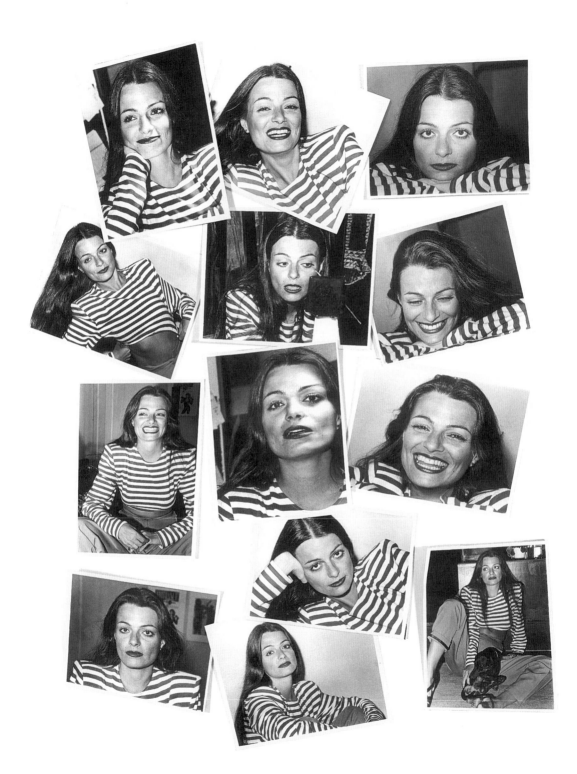

Thirty is so major. It reveals your character and starts to define your ability to mature and move on to adulthood with powerful experiences that help you realize your ability to take on life's challenges.

I know from years of being around women transitioning through thirty that each and every one of you has your own story, your time to be faced with grown-up decisions. I am convinced that how you decide to go through this passage is very much how you will approach the years ahead.

It is not a coincidence that women feel the pressure of society's clock regarding marriage and children at this time. This stress comes from loved ones and peers and their concern for you—perhaps not wanting you to be alone, and wanting you to be like everyone else. Well, we are all on a different schedule, and I believe we are meant to travel our own road, not adopt outdated ideas about the life cycle of a woman.

The dating field changes in your thirties, and some say it gets thinner. I don't agree, because you have a better sense of self and you are a better judge of what you want and who meets that standard. This is how you will attract the person you deserve.

There is so much work to do personally in your thirties. Now is the time to focus on creating good habits. Practice the Three Pillars of a healthy lifestyle: sleep, diet, and exercise. Be strong and empowered by your mind-body awareness. Open yourself up to learning about people. Be curious. Explore worlds you don't know. In your community and beyond, there is a connection you should be making, and the only way it will happen is by feeling good about yourself and having the confidence to reach out.

The secret is to just keep developing and nurturing your true, authentic self. The benefit of self-esteem is that you do everything better when you have a healthy sense of who you are. When you are practicing self-care and self-love, it is subliminally transmitted to others. Messaging self-respect attracts respect. My feeling is the more you work on yourself—your mind, body, dreams—the more you raise the bar for the type of people you attract.

Dating services offer another option for meeting people, but only if you treat them like a job interview where you are the one hiring, and the candidate must deserve the fit, healthy person you are in mind, body, and spirit. As you read this, you know I am right. A confident woman will draw the best to her. Women with insecurities send out a message that often attracts negative people and behavior.

If you are seeing someone, it is important not to feel this may be the last person on Earth for you and that you must hold on longer than you should. Not every relationship is meant to go on forever, but you do benefit from the positives and the negatives of every relationship. I was single and met someone who inspired me in many ways creatively and in business. He remains a dear friend today. I learned so much about my potential in this relationship, and I am forever grateful.

As you work on yourself, it's important to understand your own pros and cons. What do you need to improve?

My shy personality needed a change. I realized that being introverted by nature was not going to work for me as an entrepreneur trying to get a business off the ground and built for ongoing success. Since I did not feel that I had the innate ability to come out of my shell on my own, I decided to mimic a friend who was upbeat, positive, and persuasive. She was the kind of person who could make things happen. She had such power with her communication skills and the way in which she engaged meaningfully with people, investing in long-lasting relationships that contributed to her own goals, and vice versa. I was impressed with the outcome and the trust she built, and I started to incorporate her style into what I was developing as my own. Adopting her approach became so personal and authentic that even writing this I am smiling about how I got here.

I am proud to say that I have long relationships with people who have been a part of my business for many years; they are my work family, and I am so grateful for the experiences we have together.

When someone is successful at what they do, take steps to learn how they made it happen. It is important to learn what they did, but equally important to make it your own.

CARRY FORWARD YOUR CURIOUS SPIRIT FROM YOUR TWENTIES. MOVE AHEAD WITH THE CONFIDENCE FROM YOUR FIRST BIG TRANSITION, EMPOWERED TO SET ELEVATED STANDARDS FOR WHO YOU ARE, WHO YOU WILL BECOME, AND WHOM YOU ATTRACT.

Thirty is a wonderful decade for personal growth. One of the most significant lessons I learned during this time was that if you tell your story and ask for help, only then do people know how they can help. In time you will be on the other end, offering help to others who are discovering their own path.

During this time, you may also notice the fine lines on your face that used to come and then go after a good night's sleep. Well, they are not going, and strands of gray hair may start appearing here and there, too. These discoveries do take your breath away for a minute, which is precisely why this is the time to take action with your health. Fortify your immune system, nurture your skin, add quality to the food you eat, and prioritize your sleep habits.

Carry forward your curious spirit from your twenties. Move ahead with the confidence from your first big transition, empowered to set elevated standards for who you are, who you will become, and whom you attract. If you are in a marriage or a relationship, the same is true. In fact, even more so. Women understand that getting lost in their partner's identity has negative consequences, especially as years go by. The positive alternative is finding the power in yourself. **NK**

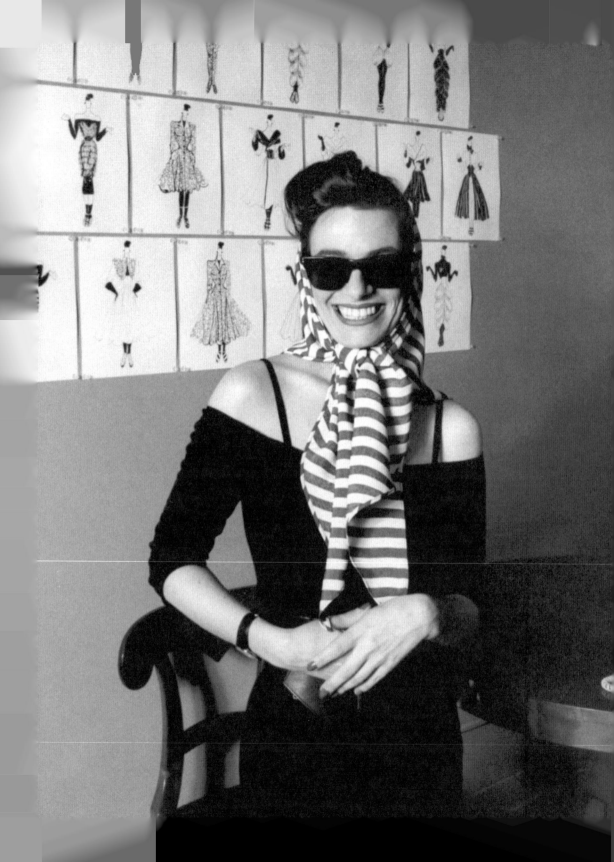

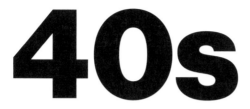

40s

FORTY BRINGS HIGH-LEVEL RESPONSIBILITIES AND
HIGH-LEVEL CHALLENGES AS YOU MAKE A NAME
FOR YOURSELF IN THE WORLD YOU CHOOSE TO CREATE.

**EXERCISE AND DIET ARE
SIGNIFICANT GAME-CHANGERS
THAT WILL EMPOWER YOU
TO BE IN CONTROL OF A LIFE
CYCLE EVERY WOMAN
EXPERIENCES DIFFERENTLY.**

While designing a swimwear collection in 1979, I thought I would make a gray sweatshirt for after a swim, which is what I wore. Sweatshirts were available in men's and boys' sizes at Army Navy stores, but the material was not typically used for clothing. When the fabric arrived, I was so excited after the first sample that I immediately made dresses, suits, gowns, coats, jackets, and tops—all with detachable shoulder pads, a cool contradiction to the gray sweats fabric. This was so much fun, and what a high to see the idea come to life. I knew the collection was touching on more than fashion; it was lifestyle.

I was so used to having my designs copied in big full-page ads by department stores that my fear once again was that I would

THIS PHOTO WITH MY SKETCHES CONFIRMS WHAT I BELIEVE TODAY:
HOW LUCKY I AM TO LIVE A CREATIVE LIFE!

present a new fashion concept only to see it reproduced by a larger company that would sell it under its brand and own it. I was struggling to pay salaries and buy fabric, and I couldn't reconcile how to protect myself.

I contacted some folks at *Women's Wear Daily* and asked for advice. They introduced me to Sidney Kimmel, who was hugely successful with Jones Apparel Group, the company he founded. We met and were in business two weeks later! The Sweats collection was bigger than anything I could have imagined. It was the perfect moment for casual, comfortable clothing for anytime—day, night, even for work. It was a new approach to style, and, *wowza*, there were lines down the block outside of stores. It was the first sportswear-inspired line worn as fashion outside the gym on the streets in everyday life.

Twelve years after I first started making clothes, I was no longer a cult underground designer. The collection went global and spurred many opportunities. Would I have realized my potential navigating the balance between artistic creativity and commerce if I had not gone off on my own?

By the time I turned forty, I was in my zone. I had countless licenses globally, including clothing for kids, shoes, hats, gloves, tights, sleepwear, you name it. My confidence and skills were in a very good place. I bought the building across the street from the space I was in and transformed it into the headquarters of the company. It housed my sample room, showroom, retail space, and offices. I worked with a project manager from an architecture firm to design the building from scratch.

I also had a concept store in SoHo for home furnishings. It was an open, loft-like space where everything was for sale, much of it one-of-a-kind or limited production. It was like walking into someone's home. I designed everything from chandeliers, metal tables, and upholstered furniture to mirrors with etchings and Japanese seed pearl bedcovers with silk sheets and comforters. I mixed in an assortment of interesting antiques and hand-crafted artisan work—anything and everything for the home. It became a place to visit in the city.

THESE PHOTOS, TAKEN FOR THE JUNE 1981 ISSUE OF *BRITISH VOGUE*, CAPTURE THE ESSENCE OF THE SWEATS COLLECTION.

TWELVE YEARS AFTER I FIRST STARTED MAKING CLOTHES, I WAS NO LONGER A CULT UNDERGROUND DESIGNER. WOULD I HAVE REALIZED MY POTENTIAL IF I HAD NOT GONE OFF ON MY OWN?

AGE WITH POWER

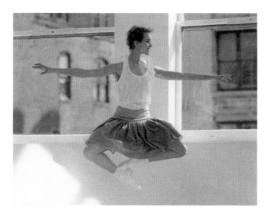

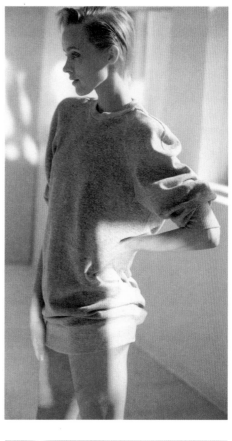

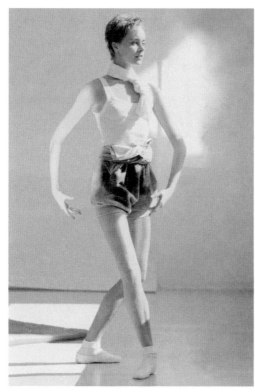

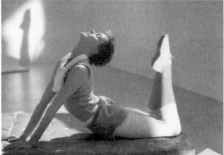

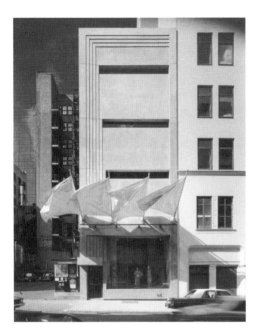

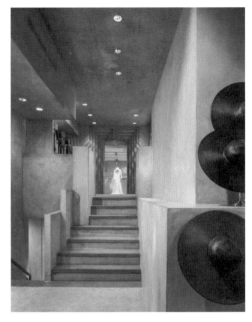

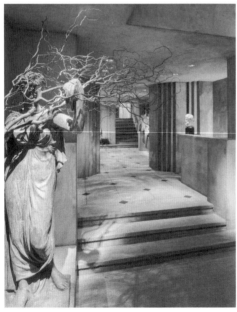

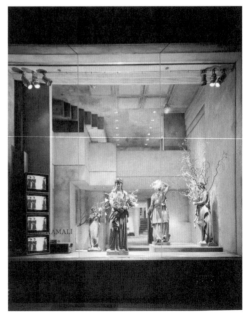

AGE WITH POWER

Unfortunately, things didn't feel right. There was global attention for my work, everything was so successful, and at this point in my career my name was recognized more than I could ever have imagined. While good press is good, I thought too much, even of a good thing, can wear thin. It felt like too much for me to live up to, and I worried that people would get bored.

Meanwhile, my Sweats collection with Jones was manufactured and sold through the license agreement, and I had no control over the distribution. They were shipping everywhere. The final straw was when I saw signs of backdoor factory shenanigans—spotting my collection sitting on rolling racks outside of discount stores on Fourteenth Street, even before it was shipped to the department stores.

Once again my self-esteem and the longevity of the company were at stake. I was faced with a decision between integrity and financial success in order to protect my brand. I had no choice but to walk away. 1986 was my last collection with Jones.

WHAT HAPPENS IN YOUR FORTIES IS YOU ARE ABLE TO MAKE THE BIG DECISIONS AND MANAGE YOUR LIFE AS A PROFESSIONAL. IT DOESN'T MEAN IT GETS EASIER; IT JUST MEANS YOU LEARN HOW TO HANDLE IT BETTER.

Now I needed to rethink my approach for how to go selective with controlled distribution. The solution came to me with an offer to make my clothes in Italy through a license with a high-end Italian company. The quality of its workmanship and the stores to which it sold—a select number of specialty stores in Europe and the United States—were regarded as the finest in the world. While the Italian company produced my luxury collection, the Japanese license I had had for many years continued the Sweats concept. Now I could regain the status of my brand and recover from the greed that had put my company and my name at risk.

What happens in your forties is you are able to make the big decisions and manage your life as a professional. It doesn't mean it gets easier; it just means you learn how to handle it better.

I had incredible confidence since achieving a level of success. I was navigating the masculine-feminine role I had to play running the business while also trying to balance having a personal life, and all while experiencing perimenopause.

As you move into your mid-forties, you are more aware of the hormonal highs and lows that affect how you feel physically, mentally, and emotionally. They are subtle and easy to ignore at first, but soon enough, they will make themselves felt. High-level responsibilities and issues become high-level challenges when the impact of menopause begins to take hold. Women do it every day, boldly and quietly, but it is difficult, to say the least. When you feel uncomfortable in your own skin, when your body and mind are experiencing changes and it seems as if everything and everyone around you is difficult, you are in an altered universe. This is real stress.

Perimenopause, the period of time when your body starts making its transition toward menopause, creeps up on you. Perhaps it's because you have been trying to delay dealing with—or even thinking about—the hot flashes, discomfort, weight gain, and mood shifts you have heard associated with this time in a woman's life. Menopause means so much more. It also reminds you that you are no longer of childbearing age. I had been saying for years, "Maybe I will adopt," but my life was so independent, the reality was that I didn't think about having children very much.

A monthly period defines so much of a woman's self-esteem, value, and femininity. Once your body starts to evolve, all of this turns upside down. Women at this time can start to feel invisible. Everything has to be done to prevent that, starting with the way you look and feel.

If you are healthy and you look good, your attitude changes. This takes discipline, but it puts you in charge of your body and your mind. It is impossible to be invisible when you have the power to manage your health and wellness.

As I moved through my forties, my search for understanding and my quest to live a balanced life expanded to finding mentors in the fields of health and well-being and educating myself as much as I could. Everywhere I went I searched for tips and ideas about healthy living. The biggest step toward my reinvention was to focus intently, taking in all of this new information and living it full-time.

Part of how I took hold of my situation was by completely rethinking my diet. I totally revamped my kitchen and ate plant-based food, tried macrobiotic

SO MANY
WONDERFUL
HOURS
EXPERIMENTING
BEHIND THE
SEWING
MACHINE.

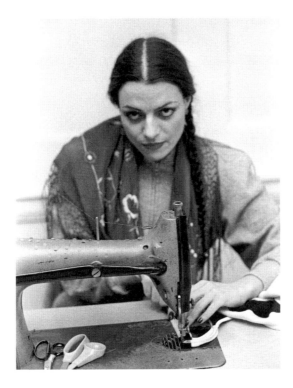

and raw, cut out sugar, and experimented with different types of fasting to see how I would feel. The dietary beliefs I was exposed to while traveling to Japan during this time—the emphasis on simple, nutritious, local ingredients tied to the seasons, the Zen sensibility—I still carry forward every day. It was in Japan that I discovered the most elegant, beautiful green teas, which are used for their calming and health benefits. I replaced coffee with antioxidant-rich green tea, and still look forward to a cup or two throughout the day.

In addition to switching to a clean diet, I worked out every day and used sleep and meditation as ways to temper the hormonal fluctuations. My metabolism was sluggish, but with the lifestyle changes I was making, I felt so balanced that when menopause was real I felt more in control.

I was listening to my body. NK

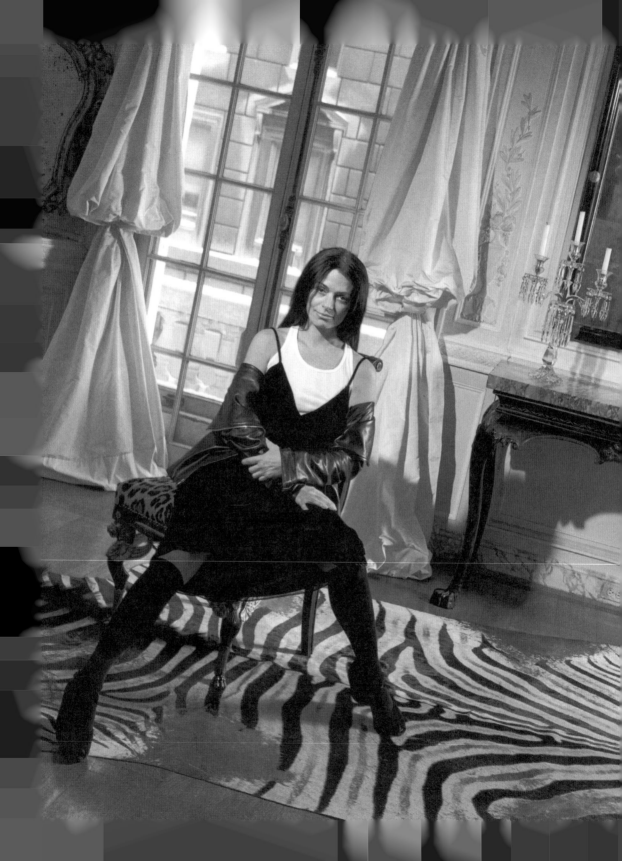

50s

TURNING FIFTY MEANS YOU HAVE SURVIVED!

THE ROLLER COASTER OF HORMONAL CHANGES WOMEN EXPERIENCE CONTINUES FOR MOST UNTIL AROUND FIFTY-FIVE, BUT IT IS BETTER UNDERSTOOD AND UNDER CONTROL. THIS IS A FREEING TIME—AN OPPORTUNITY TO TRY ADVENTURE AND TO REALIZE UNFULFILLED DREAMS AND DESIRES.

Fifty is major because now is the time for reinvention! For me, this meant a life cleanse.

My home at the time was in a town house off Fifth Avenue across from Central Park. I remember passing these beautiful buildings as a girl on my way to the museum. I grew up near the East River on Seventy-Seventh Street in Manhattan, and when it rained we would buy brownies and head for the Met. The town houses were so beautiful. The detail, the quality, just captured my imagination. I would peer into the windows to try to get a peek at what they looked like inside, conjuring the glamorous movies of the thirties and forties and picturing Cary Grant walking through the rooms.

I THOUGHT HAVING AN ELABORATE HOME WAS A DREAM COME TRUE UNTIL I REALIZED IT WASN'T, AND THAT MY POSSESSIONS WERE LIMITING MY CREATIVE SPIRIT.

When my business went global, in my mid-forties, and I was coincidentally looking for an apartment, my accountant recommended I buy something. At first I resisted because I was still in the mindset of "Can I afford it?" but then I started to look around and this amazing opportunity presented itself! There was a town house exactly where I would gaze and dream as a girl, with two owners who were both selling their spaces inside. Believe it or not, the building had been part of the Woolworth estate, and Cary Grant, who was briefly married to Woolworth heiress Barbara Hutton, had lived in the building. *Whaaaat!*

I restored the spaces and connected the two apartments into one. I made special furniture and chandeliers and collected interesting antiques and things of extreme beauty for the three floors. My design aesthetic at the time was best exemplified by my kitchen, with its eighteen-foot ceilings and one hundred silver trays running up the walls. I hung paintings of women from all eras and painting styles. I created a visual masterpiece and tribute to the space. There was beautiful detail everywhere—every fantasy of my childhood dreams. A winding marble staircase opened to a magical environment upstairs: an observatory of all glass in which to relax, meditate, and sketch. Simply wonderful.

One day as I was sitting at a lovely vintage table sketching my collection, I kept staring around the room, overwhelmed with the beauty. I felt uneasy and uncomfortable and found myself locked into a place that was not allowing me space to move forward creatively or spiritually. I needed change.

I thought seriously about moving out of the apartment and letting go of everything. I shocked myself by how much the idea actually excited me.

Every year, a friend of mine who is an astrologer would send me to a different city for my birthday. As I was turning fifty, she directed me to Madras, India (now known as Chennai). Her reading of my chart was as if she were reading my mind. She said, "You are going to let go of everything and do a life cleanse." And I said, *Yessss!* I felt so inspired to do this. I set up my plans to be in Madras on June 27, my birthday.

My friends in India happened to be part of an artists' community, and they put together a dinner under the stars. A large table of wonderful people celebrating my big birthday. As a gift, they sent me off the next morning to a

Brahman priest to have my astrological chart done, India-style. Three hours farther south at the end of June means we were getting closer to the equator, and it was hot! We arrived, and, standing in heat so dense you could actually see it, as if it were steam rising from a stove, stood a man with the darkest skin and the skinniest body, a white sarong wrapped around his hips. He stood by a hut, feeding the birds and small animals that hovered around him. He invited me into his home, which had a mud floor and very little furniture—simple and hot. The minute he began to speak, I no longer felt the heat and was captivated by his philosophical approach to astrology. Bottom line, he said, "You are ready for a life cleanse, and when you do it, it will change your life."

SHE SAID, "YOU ARE GOING TO LET GO OF EVERYTHING AND DO A LIFE CLEANSE." AND I SAID, *YESSSS!*

I returned home and put the house on the market. I contacted Christie's and organized an auction. I started to think about the two warehouses full of furniture and the samples from my fashion collections (twenty thousand pieces) I had saved from each season since I had been on my own. I had endless collections of things. I gave chalices and silver trays to St. Patrick's Cathedral. I donated antiques and a series of books on old New York to Gracie Mansion. I contributed a big art book collection to a group for AIDs and gave away and sold the furniture and all other possessions. I had three vintage cars, which I gave to people who were instrumental in my career.

I was free of my possessions and so light, so clear about the next direction in my life.

I moved into a space overlooking the Hudson River in the West Village and made a vow that going forward, I would pass on anything I wasn't using or that didn't have a purpose. I did this with books and cassette tapes for quite some time. I painted everything white in my new apartment. I painted my entire headquarters at 11 West Fifty-Sixth Street white, inside and out. It was a clean new beginning with a look to the future and all my imagination could create!

Everything in my life had played itself out and felt stale and uninspired, including a long quasi-relationship. Change was happening and welcome but nonetheless, at times, bittersweet. I was filled with excitement, as well as a bit of fear of the unknown, but that passed within a short time.

As a result of the research I had done and the trailblazing experts I was lucky to meet as I sought out more information, my philosophy about leading a healthy and fit life was now so much more informed.

THE WELLNESS CAFÉ WAS THE BEGINNING OF MY OUTWARD COMMITMENT TO A HEALTHY LIFESTYLE.

Dr. Andrew Weil introduced me to his proactive, natural approach to wellness and preventative medicine. Native American medicine woman Dr. Tieraona Low Dog opened my mind to the magic that comes from the earth, inspiring me to incorporate traditional remedies from herbs and plants into my life. Author Michael Pollan, an early voice in the conversation about the food we eat and how it is farmed, created a narrative that gave me guidelines for making better choices when it came to my diet.

There was so much wisdom to digest and implement. I amped up my efforts as I transitioned through postmenopausal hormonal activity.

I was working out at Radu, a circuit training system developed by a Romanian Olympic trainer, alternating it with a rigorous Pilates practice. I felt better about my body than ever in my life. Physically and emotionally I was balanced and steady, with no hormonal upsets. The more I stayed on point with my diet and exercise plan, the better I felt, and the better I slept, which is critical for daily restoration. Could it be that post-menopause, post-fifty, I was better than ever?

The relief of not having hormones ruling your life makes room for clear thinking and emotional calm. Because I was staying fit and feeling good about my body, I was actually freer and more expressive in relation to my femininity and womanhood than before.

I am here to testify that you can feel better and be better with age.

My confidence and my humor about life have become more free-spirited as I have gotten older.

I AM HERE TO TESTIFY THAT YOU CAN FEEL BETTER AND BE BETTER WITH AGE.

I am less angry about even the things that deserve an angry response. My self-esteem empowers me to behave with a more open mind. I am kinder and more generous. Generosity is easy because you realize how much you have, and therefore you have nothing to lose.

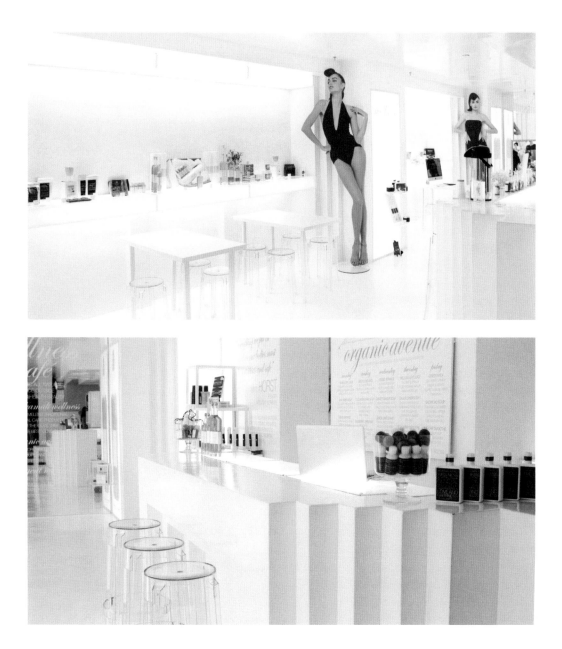

Midway through my fifties, after 9/11, I met a guy at a Yankees game during the World Series. We started talking about olive oil! He was from Barcelona and wanted to bring the best olive oils in the world to the States. Growing up with a Lebanese mother and a Basque father, we used olive oil for everything. My mother used it in our food, on our hair to keep it shiny, on our skin to hydrate and protect, as a supplement to keep us regular, and on and on. As an adult, I continued the tradition and was obsessed with olive oil products, especially the raw olive oil soaps and cleansers I would order from everywhere. By the last game of the series, he suggested we go on the hunt together! *What?* I am the most regimented person you'll ever meet—not known to be spontaneous, especially while running a business and producing four collections a year. I thought, *Never*.

Well, in March he contacted me and I actually had time to go on this exploratory adventure. I met him in Barcelona, and off we went driving south through Spain's endless farms and olive orchards up through the south of France and through Italy, sourcing the best oils along the Mediterranean olive belt. We ended our expedition in Milan, where we developed the packaging for a line we called Olive You.

The olive orchards changed my life in so many ways. The trip fit perfectly with the years of research I had done about leading a healthy lifestyle. And here I was with a handsome younger man. It blossomed into an all-encompassing experience of mind, body, and soul.

I discovered over the years that younger men are frequently attracted to women who are confident and older, and I think there is something to an experience like this. When you are strong and self-assured, there is a sort of comfort men find in a more free-spirited approach to a relationship. There is less pressure to think about marriage, kids, commitment, and responsibilities; it is just about the experience. It is a win-win for all.

I was feeling great and incredibly empowered. My spirit reflected my appearance, and my appearance reflected my spirit. This is what happens when you make room in your life for curiosity and adventure: Doors open to worlds you never imagined.

The Wellness Café, which I started at my flagship building in New York soon after returning from the olive oil adventure, emerged as a way for me to start sharing my story about health and well-being with others. Bringing attention to products and practices that help boost the immune system and form the foundation of a healthy lifestyle had become a motivation and purpose for me following the events of 9/11. A new level of stress was reaching everyone, and a strong immune system would be more important than ever. I brought in the organic olive oils and personal care products derived from the orchards. I created scents from the different regions I had visited that embodied wellness, including lavender from France, orange flower from Italy, jasmine from Spain. The Wellness Café was a place where folks could come try different remedies and recipes. It became a hub for teas, talks, films, classes, and meditation.

The reinvention I experienced in my fifties also extended to beauty and the evolution of my personal style. This was my decade of red hair. It was a look I had never considered before, but I loved every minute of it and gained so much from living outside of my box.

I stopped wearing makeup, too. I was aware of changes in the texture of my skin in my late thirties and more so in my forties, when little lines started appearing. They stayed and became part of the expression of my face. As I approached fifty, I was no longer happy wearing foundation. It never completely matched my skin tone, and actually made my fine lines more visible. I had a license agreement with Warner Cosmetics at the time, and I came up with a skin care concept that allowed for a fresh, foundation-free face.

The idea of not having to hide your skin is very liberating. It transformed my attitude and sense of myself. Imagine not caring about the lighting in a room or on an elevator. Imagine working out, sweating, making love, and your bare skin is glowing.

For me, showing my skin, lines and all, was an honest and authentic expression of my best self. It showed that I was not trying to hide my age and that I didn't feel insecure about who I was and who I was becoming.

I encourage you all to welcome the reinvention that can lead to the best time of your life. This is what it means to age with power.   NK

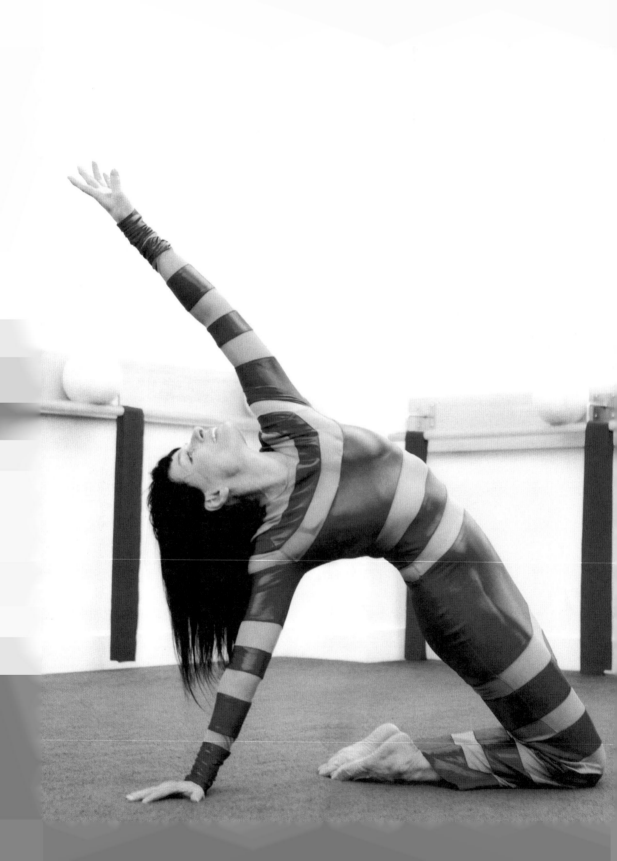

60s

TURNING SIXTY IS AMAZING IF YOU HAVE BEEN WORKING ON FITNESS, HEALTH, AND SELF-NURTURING.

I NEVER THOUGHT I WAS MEANT TO HAVE A SOUL MATE, BUT TO MY SURPRISE, I MET MINE AT SIXTY-FIVE!

My curiosity and open approach to new endeavors continues today, and it was certainly expressed in full force in my sixties. I had meetings as usual with interesting business opportunities, and in those meetings I was always impressed with the incredible people I met. In one meeting, I had a great connection with a forward-thinking leader, and as fate would have it, he moved to Walmart a year later and contacted me to come meet with him. I told him I had never been to a Walmart, and he said, "Now you will come and see for yourself," so of course I went.

STRETCH, MOVE, AND DON'T STOP.

I have always been a Sam Walton fan. His story is truly one of success and American spirit. It was moving to see how they had memorialized his very simple, understated life at the company headquarters with a museum-like setup of his office and pickup truck. Walking through the superstore I was amazed by the quantity and quality of affordable products for anything one might need.

Their team wanted to take a stab at fashion and thought I might be a match. I was not sure it was a fit, as I believe that for a budget-conscious shopper, classic style is more enduring than seasonal fashion. I left a newspaper clipping on the conference table of a simple white shirtdress and said that this, to me, was what fashion at Walmart should embody: timeless essentials that would have real meaning for their customer.

A year or two later I received another call. They reconsidered my suggestion and offered to come meet me in my studio to talk about my original concept. We made a deal, and I created a line for Walmart using their suppliers (which, by the way, make high-end clothing, as well). I asked lots of questions about their shopper and created a closet of the core styles I thought anyone, anywhere, would need for any situation: a white shirt, a trench, a little black dress, a great-fitting black pant, cargo pants, and T-shirts, which were a big hit. I even designed shoes, including a great pump, a loafer, and ballet slippers. Everything was priced under $20! It was the same fit and design I've always done for my clients, but because the volume was so large, we were able to make it all at a great price. We launched in stores and online. Walmart discovered customers who had never shopped there before buying the collection. Smart entrepreneurs were buying in bulk and selling the items on eBay for two hundred dollars apiece.

A wonderful result of the partnership was that it gave me a new opportunity to continue my work with the public school system. I am a public school graduate and because of the scholarships and grants I received, I was able to have an extended education. As a teen, I was a student at Washington Irving High School, a girls' school near Fourteenth Street I chose because

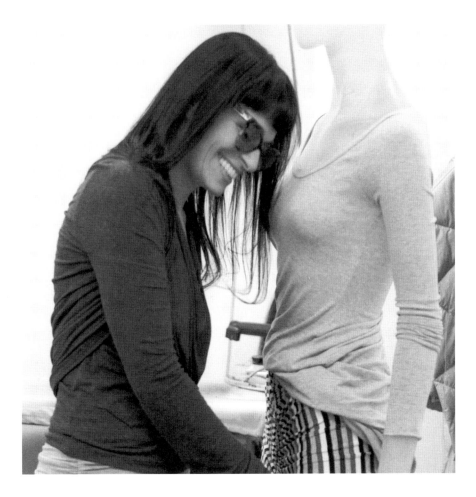

I LOVE MY JOB.

I'd heard it had a great art department. It was a tough school back then, and when I was contacted by the principal in the late eighties, the school was by that time coed, but let's just say that the four metal detectors in the entrance indicated it was still a tough place. I volunteered to mentor a class, and created a fashion studio in my old homeroom—room 741. I have been working with New York City's schools ever since.

When I signed the Walmart agreement, I consciously thought about the teachers and parents in our country's public school system. I'd noticed that some moms would not go to parent-teacher meetings because they did not feel they had appropriate clothes to meet their children's teachers. Now I had great-fitting, well-made clothing for Mom and her budget. And for the teachers, I felt they needed a wardrobe of suits and dresses that created dignified space in the classroom, allowing them to dress up for work. I spoke to Randi Weingarten, president of the American Federation of Teachers, and she invited me to do a fashion show featuring teachers at their annual conference in Detroit.

This wonderful experience with Walmart taught me the value of style at a price and the democracy of fashion. It also reinforced what I believed: that e-commerce was where it was at. Online shopping was where I was going, and today, I primarily sell to online accounts, as

STAY RELEVANT IN EVERY WAY, AND YOU WILL KEEP GROWING, LEARNING, AND FEELING EMPOWERED. IF YOU FEEL GOOD AND LOOK GOOD, YOUR ACTUAL AGE MAKES NO DIFFERENCE FOR ALL YOU ARE ABLE TO DO.

well as from my own website. My department store business is focused online, and as a result I have been able to ride through the disruption the fashion industry has experienced. Early on, Walmart was also embracing sustainability in order to be a responsible global supplier, and imposed regulations on all suppliers to meet their requirements. I thank them for all they do and for everything I learned from them.

My love of technology really expanded during my sixties. E-commerce and new forms of communication became my obsession. This was an expansive time for me. I learned all I could about innovations in augmented reality, virtual reality, and artificial intelligence, and how to incorporate these modalities into my business.

While the 1960s were a time of revolution I was lucky to experience, I feel that we are now in the midst of an even bigger revolution fueled by our connection through technology. In an instant, we can connect across a room or across the globe.

Exploring the new world and staying curious has to be a part of who you are in order to be involved today. Fear of the unknown is real, but the faster you learn, the more access there will be to jobs, and even volunteer opportunities. It is important to ask for help if you need it. I recommend asking folks older than your grandchildren, who have more patience, to show you the ropes. You deserve respect—get it from someone fifty-plus!

I have tried to hire women in their sixties, but a fear of technology often limits their ability to fit into a business environment that relies on technologic fluency. Companies need the stability, experience, and wisdom of people who are post-fifty, but it can be difficult to find talented people who are not challenged by a simple Excel chart. Stay relevant in every way, and you will keep growing, learning, and feeling empowered. If you feel good and look good, your actual age makes no difference for all you are able to do.

Working out every day is as important as it was during menopause. Finding a class you like—barre, Pilates, Gyrokinesis, yoga, or anything else you discover you like—should be part of your daily plan. It should be something you look forward to and that makes you feel good. I find routine is always good for fitness; I try to set aside the same time every day so my body expects to exercise.

an Schrager has been my dear friend since the days of Studio 54. He started New York's most legendary nightclub with his college friend Steve Rubell in 1976, and went on to completely transform the nightlife and hospitality industries. We met when he asked me to create a costume for Grace Jones to wear for her performance for Studio's big New Year's Eve party in 1977. I designed a cutout gold draped gown over a shimmering bodysuit that contrasted her glowing skin and impeccably fit body. From then on, Ian's staff dated my staff; Steve and the doormen who presided outside wore my Sleeping Bag Coats (and so did folks hoping to get in, thinking it would help). It was a brief but intense electric moment in time that left a lasting legacy that has yet to be repeated. Ian has been a friend, a mentor, and a source of support and inspiration. I hope I have been some of that for him, as well. He is my family.

As any family member might, Ian expressed deep concern over some of the men I had been with in my life. He was certainly not shy about sharing his feelings. He had never introduced me to anyone, so I never expected the invitation to meet a man he knew. "Hey, Norm, there's a guy I want you to meet!" I thought for sure it was for a business opportunity, but he said, "No, no, this is a guy for *you*!" Shocking! I was actually a little concerned about who he would think was the guy "for me," but he was so right, and is responsible for having introduced me to my soul mate. At sixty-five!

The funny thing . . . is a flashback to 1970:

For my twenty-fifth birthday, a friend gave me the gift of a reading with an astrologer. I went to see this woman who proceeded to do my entire life chart. Her reading of my childhood was so precise and detailed it was powerful. Then she looked into the future and talked about my career and the various plateaus I would reach during different times in my life.

"In your sixties," she said, "you will move up another level to a new place in your career and, oh, you will meet your soul mate when you are *sixty-five*!"

"Slit my wrists," I replied. "What are you saying—*sixty-five*?!?!"

AGE WITH POWER

"IN YOUR SIXTIES," SHE SAID, "YOU WILL MOVE UP ANOTHER LEVEL TO A NEW PLACE IN YOUR CAREER AND, OH, YOU WILL MEET YOUR SOUL MATE WHEN YOU ARE *SIXTY-FIVE*!"

"Yes," she said, softening the blow, "that is when you will be ready."

Even though I was determined to prove her wrong, I failed to do so. I forgot about the prediction and adjusted to being the one who doesn't have a life partner, but has great friends and interesting relationships instead. And I must say I was comfortable with that, especially post-menopause, my hormones no longer playing with me.

I am sure that timing had everything to do with meeting my soul mate. He had been a family guy in the suburbs with three kids. That would never have worked for me. He sees photos of me with red hair and his eyes cross, so clearly that wouldn't have worked for him. Well, I definitely needed that red hair period, so the timing worked out for both of us. We met at a point in our lives when we both felt so secure about who we were that we could give of ourselves in a way that is as close to unconditional as you can get. We are evolved enough to be open to all friendships and relationships, never eliminating anyone from our circle of friends. We have passion for our work and we admire and respect each other on the highest level. The adventure we live is because we have the same moral compass, and that comes from age, experience, and appreciation. We both feel gratitude for having met our soul mate during this lifetime, and we know that every day is special for us to have with each other. **NK**

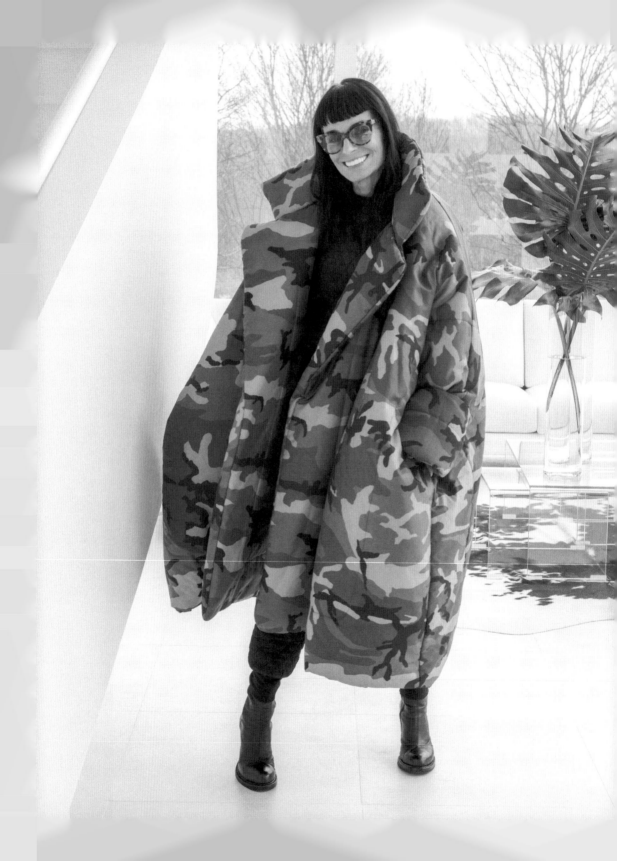

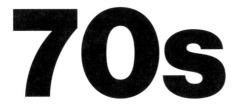

70s

WHO KNEW THAT SEVENTY COULD BE THE MOST ACTIVE AND EXCITING DECADE YET? CONTINUE ACHIEVING YOUR GOALS AND SETTING NEW ONES.

THIS IS THE POWER OF AGE.

I am seventy-five and older than ninety percent of the people I know. Spiritually, I identify as at least twenty years younger, just with more experience! Not only do I feel that much younger, but quite frankly I am treated that way by most people who do not know my age.

Whenever I do say my age, and that I met my soul mate at sixty-five, women, especially younger women, want to know more. I am presenting a narrative that does not fit the one most of us have been led to believe is the predestined plan for women.

It is impossible for every woman to expect that the partner she is meant to have will appear by the time she reaches thirty. It certainly didn't for me. My plan did not include any of the expiration dates we are fed regarding marriage, kids, and career.

I HAVE WORN A SLEEPING BAG COAT EVERY WINTER SINCE I MADE THE FIRST ONE AFTER A CAMPING TRIP IN 1974.

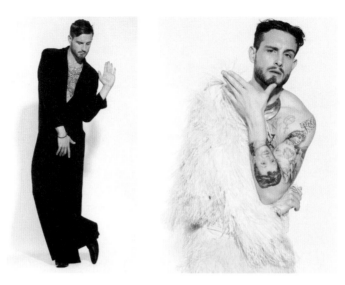

FLUID STYLE, WHICH WAS PROMINENT IN THE SEVENTIES, BLURRED GENDER LINES AND ENCOURAGED FULL EXPRESSION. WHAT A WELCOME RETURN.

The partner for you may not materialize when you think he or she should, or may never appear, and that cannot be how you define your life. Relationships of all kinds are important and serve a purpose for your personal development, as mine did for me.

Now is the time to have open, candid conversations about age. Not about aging gracefully in submission or becoming invisible. Now is the time to talk about aging with power, purpose, and a newly defined authentic beauty.

I feel that because I consciously worked on a healthy lifestyle I have been in a good place since transitioning through my forties and fifties. After fifty-five, you are no longer at the mercy of your hormones. You are wiser as a result of countless life lessons.

My seventies fit my plan and my purpose. My goal has always been to lead a creative life and to make women feel good about themselves.

I have been introduced as an "aging guru" and a "wellness goddess," and my first inclination was to just laugh out loud, but then I thought, *Why shouldn't I be happy to share what I have learned about wellness and aging?* So here I am in my seventies, fully exploring how I can further manifest my purpose.

AGE WITH POWER

There is no beauty product or substitute for a healthy lifestyle. To this day I incorporate the Three Pillars: sleep, diet and exercise. I meditate regularly, I practice intermittent fasting, and I try to balance an incredibly stressful schedule with self-care.

I never thought about my chronological age or even talked about it until this book because I so did not connect in any way to the number. That age represented someone retired, checked out, or slowing down.

Well, I have dreams I want to realize and ideas that fit the times in which we are living. I am busier than I can ever remember. It is so hard to say no to exciting new projects.

NOW IS THE TIME TO HAVE OPEN, CANDID CONVERSATIONS ABOUT AGE. NOT ABOUT AGING GRACEFULLY IN SUBMISSION OR BECOMING INVISIBLE. NOW IS THE TIME TO TALK ABOUT AGING WITH POWER, PURPOSE, AND A NEWLY DEFINED AUTHENTIC BEAUTY.

I am in a business in complete disruption, as are many others outside of the fashion industry. When there is disruption, the status quo no longer works. You must change or disappear.

My interest in technology—from VR to AR and AI—excites every part of me. I think if I weren't a fashion designer, I would have loved this world of invention and the future. My mind soars with ideas about what can be achieved that hasn't been done before, and I am in talks with folks about seeing these ideas come to fruition.

Thanks to an early move to e-commerce, I am happy to say that my company is in sync with the times, and this achievement gives me the opportunity to do more things I love, like continuing to collaborate with my dear friend Twyla Tharp on dance costumes for the American Ballet Theatre, designing furniture, creating innovation in fashion and beauty, and working on how wellness practices can become more democratic and inclusive.

Several years ago, I started presenting my collection on both women and men. This approach to fashion, which I now believe is one of the most directional influences of our time, came about naturally. An assistant hairdresser was really excited about the clothes while we were photographing the collection. He was in a total New York Dolls getup, and I asked if he knew them. He said yes, and he knew that I dressed them back in the seventies—back when my clothes were initially designed for women, but fifty percent of my clients were in fact men. I told him that after the shoot he could try some of the clothes on and we would photograph him, too. I posted the pictures on social media and noticed quite a positive response. At this time, I also noticed nonbinary celebrities and models styled wearing my clothes at events and in the press. I decided from that shoot onward that we would always present a gender-fluid vision of the collection, to both press and buyers, and on our website. We relabeled the clothing with sizing based on body type to show that the pieces were for everyone. I am so happy to say that clothes no longer define the person—now the person defines the clothes.

The Wellness Café concept continues to be a source of inspiration and purpose for me, and I have rethought what I think it should mean today. Last year I launched a new personal care brand based on safe, timeless ingredients and sustainable packaging and practices. It is a range for all men and women that supports a healthy lifestyle and is not about fads or excess. It is called NORMALIFE, which, yes, also means a normal life! A normal life today entails a balanced, less stressful, sustainable approach to living based on simple ingredients that work.

I don't think about staying relevant; I just think about what people need that is important, and that makes me relevant.

I have discovered the power of age. I look at it positively, and I continuously work on feeling good about myself. Phrases like "age-appropriate," "anti-wrinkle," and "anti-age" aren't in my vocabulary. I hope that people will start feeling good about their age and understand that youthful beauty is wonderful, but very short-lived. In fact, beauty through the decades can be redefined, especially when we are doing all we can to live well.

Because of my desire to lead a creative life and to live my purpose, my outlook and approach must remain positive and inspired.

I am the author of my dream.

I have the ability to live this dream because I am doing my best to take care of my body, which in turn supports my mind. A sense of humor and a positive attitude about every new day make it fun. It is so important to start the healthy lifestyle protocol early, or at least to start immediately, so we can all age with power and be the authors of our dreams. NK

AGE WITH POWER

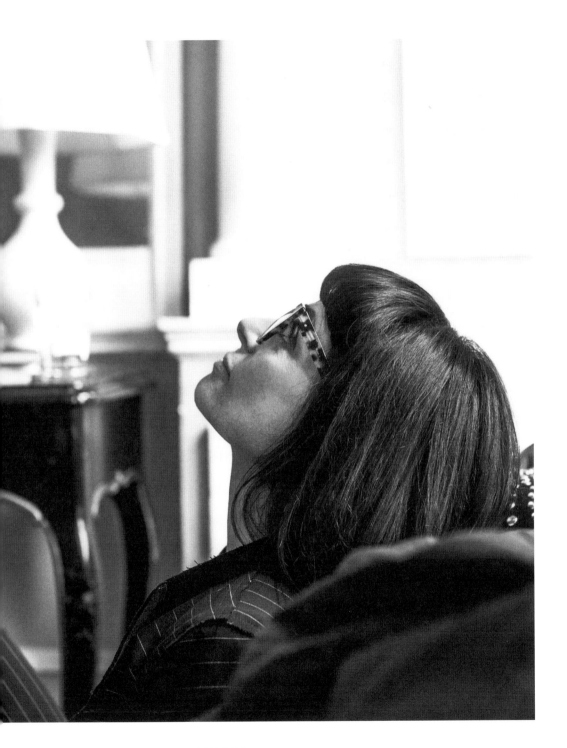

THE DECADES | 70s

80s, 90s... 100

STAY HEALTHY, FIT, AND INSPIRED, AND KEEP PUSHING FORWARD TO ENJOY EVERY OUNCE OF THE LIFE YOU HAVE CREATED.

When I was in my twenties, I envisioned what I would look like at sixty. I assumed I would be wearing a bun, sort of Georgia O'Keeffe–style, with a black dress. I would let age happen to me. I know now that working on living a healthy lifestyle adds another layer of agility, attitude, and spirit that has helped me define my productivity and relevance.

It's clear that chronological age—the number of years a person has been alive—and biological age—how old a person seems—are very different things. Especially since biological age is deeply impacted by lifestyle factors, and the concept of what chronological age looks like is based on antiquated visual references.

We are always surprised by how much younger everyone looks than their actual age, so clearly we need to be more forthcoming about age so that we become familiar with what thirty/forty/fifty/sixty/seventy and beyond really look like *today*. Yes, I think we should ask people, especially women, how old they are, and share our own age, as well.

I am very much aware of the fear of being aged out by your chronological age for a position you want or currently hold, or for your desirability as a date. Every time I ask a woman her age, it takes time for her to reply, as if she is never asked and hasn't quite decided how to answer.

Aging with power will change these objectifying myths. I believe looking good, feeling good, and having experience is a mighty combination.

The misconceptions and misnomers attached to aging are associated with a number of tag phrases that are no longer acceptable: "You look good for your age" and—my favorite—when I am with my partner walking arm in arm or hugging and we are told "how cute" we are! Age is the last bastion where discrimination is still acceptable. The beauty and fashion industries campaign against it with anti-aging products and airbrushing, and we see it fueled by social media's feature-blurring filters.

Youth can no longer remain the only definition of beauty. There is an attitude, a confidence, and a beauty that comes with age, which cannot be found in youth. It is about body language and a sense of power and calm, and it is appealing (especially to younger men for some reason).

Seventy is what I know at this time. I am at the upper end of baby boomers, so I don't have many women in the modern generation (postwar) to look to for examples. I feel I can be a representative who is not a celebrity with a glam squad to keep me looking good "for my age"! My beauty secret is not about the makeup, the beauty tips, the Spanx, the hair extensions, or the lashes. My beauty secret is to be authentic and to follow simple personal care practices. Be fit and glow, and anything you wear will look great.

There are inspiring women in their eighties, nineties, and beyond who stay active and relevant. An observation I've made about the women I admire in this age group is that they all have one thing in common: Every single one of them still dances. Dancing is everything. It is full of spirit and joy. Once you hear the music, you start moving. You can't go back and edit. I believe that what keeps people going is their effort to actively enjoy every moment of their life.

I discovered a woman on Instagram named Tao Porchon-Lynch, a 101-year-old yoga instructor. She was moving her body every day, dressing up and doing her hair and makeup with, I am sure, the same delight she had at twenty-seven. (I must add she inspired me to incorporate yoga into my exercise practice.) Reflecting on the beauty of nature (while dressed in a gown and doing a graceful side plank), Tao noted in one Instagram post, "Even the trees get more beautiful as they age."

I contacted Tao to ask if she would share some of her wisdom. She told me she began each morning early, watching the sunrise. "I look outside my window to the sky and tell myself that this is going to be the best day of my life," she said. "Whatever you put in your mind materializes. So materialize what you want to happen and know that it's possible." The key to long life, she added, is positive thinking. "I don't feel any different now that I've passed one hundred. I'm not even scared. And I will never stop practicing yoga."

AGE WITH POWER

AN OBSERVATION I'VE MADE ABOUT THE WOMEN I ADMIRE IN THIS AGE GROUP IS THAT THEY ALL HAVE ONE THING IN COMMON:

EVERY SINGLE ONE OF THEM STILL DANCES.

DANCING IS EVERYTHING.

I am reading more and more about longevity and interviewing scientists who study this topic, as well. There is documentation that we can live to one hundred twenty. Inspired by Tao, I have decided I want that to be my goal! I believe that if you aim high with anything you do, you then make a daily commitment toward reaching that dream.

This keeps me focused regarding how I lead my life and inspires me to make better choices. My thought is, if I fall short of my goal, at least I made an effort to get as far as I was meant to go. Each day that I work out, eat right, and feel proud of what I accomplished gives me a great sense of satisfaction. A good night's sleep seems to come along with it, and meditation is the anchor for that. Connecting to people with kindness is so uplifting and helps share positive energy. Hug and cuddle with your dog, embrace folks you meet, and cherish those you love. Sing, dance, and laugh every chance you get.

I want to make the most of this lifetime, and I am purposely making an effort to do so. **NK**

STYLE

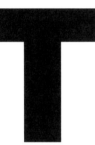

The one thing I am sure of, and I learned with experience, is that style survives fashion and personal style is developed with time. The path to developing personal style is an adventure. As kids, we wear all the things we love, sometimes all at the same time. We don't think about how it looks together; we love every piece of clothing that makes us happy. Then we start being influenced by friends, peer pressure, magazines, popular culture, and, these days, social media. During this period of time, every trend, label, new fad, or movement is part of our fashion experiment. As we learn more about ourselves and define who we are and who we want to be, we narrow the selection of trends we want to follow—or we create our own. The more you know who you are as you move through your life, the more you develop your personal style. This is when you manifest the full expression of your individuality and convey it to the world, in part through your clothes. Cultivating personal style means that every piece of clothing you own will have a purpose in your wardrobe.

The decades of fashion trends I have seen come and go enable me to appreciate the styles that remain relevant and appealing over the years. Women who understand the value of timeless style look amazing all the time. Think about Audrey Hepburn, Jackie Kennedy, Lena Horne. They wore the clothes and defined their style, not the other way around.

THE PATH TO DEVELOPING PERSONAL STYLE IS AN ADVENTURE.

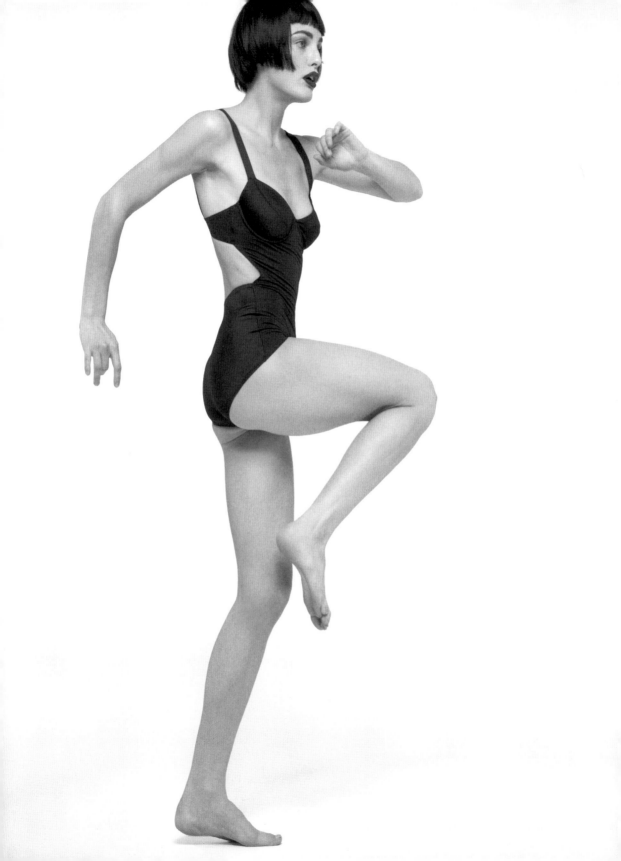

was indoctrinated into fashion at an early age. Making beautiful clothing for me was among my mother's many talents. She was prolific. Every day I had a new outfit. Well, actually, sometimes she had me make multiple outfit changes in a single day, and, yes, she photographed them. She created an album called "Norma's Life in Pictures"! It was her lookbook of children's outfits. She created detailed coats and dresses fit for a princess, inspired by British royalty and meticulously researched. All designed for me to model. She did my hair; she had hats and great little shoes, the works. I must admit that as a result of the daily posing I was camera-shy for forty years!

As I grew into my teens and my own sensibilities developed, I began to want clothes my mother wouldn't make for me. Our tastes were so different. She preferred my hair in a pageboy bob; I wanted to tease it three feet high. She veered toward formal Chesterfield coats and traditional tweeds; I longed for skinny pants. So, inspired by her example, I started to make clothing myself. My specialty was going to S. Klein, a discount department store on Fourteenth Street around the corner from my high school, where I would buy dresses from the two-dollar table, take them home, and deconstruct them. Magic! I also made intricate tops out of scarves by draping the fabric lots of different ways and holding it all together with hidden safety pins. I was sixteen! I didn't know how to attach zippers, so I would sew myself into capri pants and carry around a seam ripper and thread.

I DIDN'T KNOW HOW TO ATTACH ZIPPERS, SO I WOULD SEW MYSELF INTO CAPRI PANTS AND CARRY AROUND A SEAM RIPPER AND THREAD.

Films from the thirties and forties offered some of my earliest influences. Gene Tierney, Katharine Hepburn, and Cary Grant embodied American style and glamour. Europe has centuries of fashion history; American fashion is new by contrast. I loved films like *The Women*, which came to epitomize the classic American style still seen on the red carpet today.

I became obsessed with wearing vintage, and eventually sold vintage pieces when we opened the first KAMALI store in 1968. This inspired my personal challenge to create designs that would become what I imagined as the vintage of the future. In 1973, I designed a collection of dresses in a jersey knit. They were conceived to be timeless, multi-style, easy fit, easy travel, easy care, and to be enjoyed for many years. Styles from that collection, like the All In One Dress, which can be worn eight different ways, are still in my line today.

I design intuitively. I don't follow trends. I don't really think about it. I love clothes that are fun to wear, that move with me and never need dry cleaning. I design from my life experience and create solutions, which is how the styles for which I am best known—like the Sweats collection and swimwear—came into being. I have been making the Sleeping Bag Coat ever since a camping trip in the seventies, after which I came home and cut up my sleeping bag to keep me warm during the winter. In the days after 9/11, we were brought back to work over a sudden demand for them, even though it was still warm outside. People were stranded in hotel lobbies and airports, and the coats became safe cocoons for so many. I love taking blankets, vintage shawls—well, just about everything—and turning them into designs to wear. I find beautiful cloth in any form and want to wear it, so needless to say, these pieces become timeless and sustainable, like the collection that started from the gift of a silk parachute.

When I was first starting out, I was quite frankly shocked that anyone would pay to buy my designs. And then, to hear that women felt empowered by the styles I had created, because they made them feel good, was even more encouraging. It was meaningful for me to understand that clothing could affect self-esteem, especially since, at that time, I was wondering what value my work had when people were finding cures for cancer and I was obsessed with the length of a hem.

Designing swimwear was a natural for me because I've always loved swimming and it followed my fine art training studying anatomy and drawing the human form. A swimsuit is either the most liberating or intimidating piece of clothing a woman wears. Reaching the place where you feel your best is a process. I've learned that a healthy, fit body is always a work in progress, and that remaining faithful to the Three Pillars of sleep, diet, and exercise is the most powerful support system we have for feeling good about how we look. The swimsuit really doesn't matter; it is how you feel in your head about your body. The way you carry yourself says everything about how you feel. This is true for anything you wear. **NK**

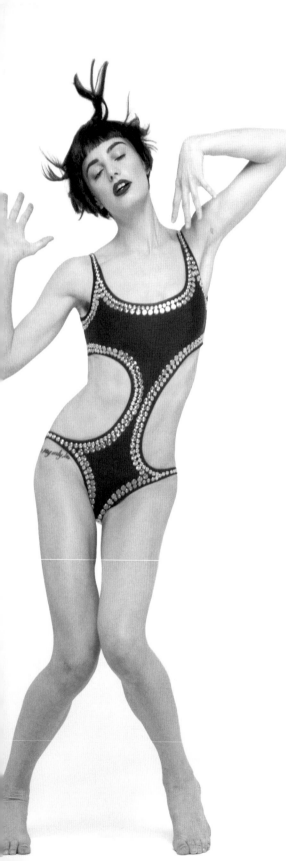

OWN YOUR STYLE AND NO ONE ELSE'S.

PUT LOOKS TOGETHER THAT MAKE YOU FEEL AS THOUGH THERE IS NOTHING YOU CAN'T DO. YOU ARE DRESSED AND **YOU ARE INVINCIBLE.**

THINK ABOUT WHAT YOU LIKE TO WEAR AND FIND THE PERFECT STYLES THAT FIT YOUR LIFE. ACCENT YOUR STYLE WITH SPECIAL ONE-OF-A-KIND ACCESSORIES OR JACKETS TO CREATE A CURATED COLLECTION OF LOOKS YOU WILL HAVE FUN WEARING. OR IGNORE THIS COMPLETELY AND DO THE OPPOSITE. BUT MAKE IT YOUR OWN.

PERSONAL STYLE IS JUST THAT... PERSONAL

IT SHOULDN'T BE WHAT YOU LIKE THAT SOMEONE ELSE IS WEARING OR A FLEETING TREND THAT JUST DOESN'T WORK FOR YOU, YOUR BODY TYPE, OR YOUR LIFESTYLE.

POWER DRESSING

REMEMBER TO WEAR A SMILE.
IT DEFUSES FEAR.

SUCCESSFUL GAME-CHANGERS LIKE STEVE JOBS, IAN SCHRAGER, AND TWYLA THARP

WEAR A UNIFORM.

IT IS BELIEVED THEY DO THIS TO ELIMINATE SMALL DECISIONS IN ORDER TO MAKE TIME FOR THE BIG IDEAS.

PERSONAL WARDROBE STYLE IS ALSO A SORT OF UNIFORM: ONE THAT REFLECTS OUR ATTITUDE AND MAKES THE IMPORTANT FIRST IMPRESSION.

DRESS SMART.

BUY CLOTHING YOU WILL REALLY WEAR.

SELECT GO-TO STYLES THAT MAKE YOU FEEL GOOD BECAUSE YOU ALWAYS LOOK GREAT IN THEM.

DON'T BUY EMOTIONALLY, BUY ONLY WHAT YOU CAN AFFORD.

PERSONAL STYLE DOESN'T COME WITH A PRICE TAG.

IT'S SO MUCH EASIER TO BUILD A WARDROBE AROUND **TIMELESS** CLOTHES THAT CAN BE **SEASONLESS** DO NOT REQUIRE DRY CLEANING AND HAVE **MULTIPLE PURPOSES**

MAKING WISE SHOPPING CHOICES IS THE MOST SUSTAINABLE THING YOU CAN DO

IN MY LIFETIME AS A DESIGNER OF WOMEN'S CLOTHING, I HAVE HEARD STORIES OVER AND OVER AGAIN OF WOMEN BUYING CLOTHES SMALLER THAN THEIR ACTUAL SIZE.

DON'T BUY CLOTHES THAT AREN'T YOUR SIZE

THE HOPE OF LOSING WEIGHT SOMEDAY TO WEAR THE STYLE IS IRRATIONAL BEHAVIOR BASED ON POOR SELF-ESTEEM, AND IT IS A COSTLY APPROACH TO BUILDING A WARDROBE. PLUS, IT MAKES YOU FEEL DISAPPOINTED EVERY TIME YOU LOOK AT THESE PIECES OR TRY THEM ON.

KEEP A MANAGEABLE, ACTIVE LIFESTYLE TO MAINTAIN YOUR HEALTHY SIZE, AND IT WILL LEAVE YOU WITH A CLOSET FULL OF CLOTHING YOU LOVE TO WEAR.

IF YOU FEEL UNCOMFORTABLE WITH A PART OF YOUR BODY, THINK ABOUT A PLAN TO CREATE A HEALTHIER, MORE FIT PHYSIQUE—AND FIT DOESN'T MEAN SKINNY! FIT CAN BE THICK OR THIN—AND THEN FOCUS ON THE POSITIVE WITH CLOTHING THAT FLATTERS.

STRIP NAKED

IN FRONT OF A FULL-LENGTH MIRROR ONCE A MONTH TO DECIDE WHAT YOU LIKE ABOUT YOURSELF AND HOW YOU CAN EMPHASIZE IT WITH YOUR WARDROBE

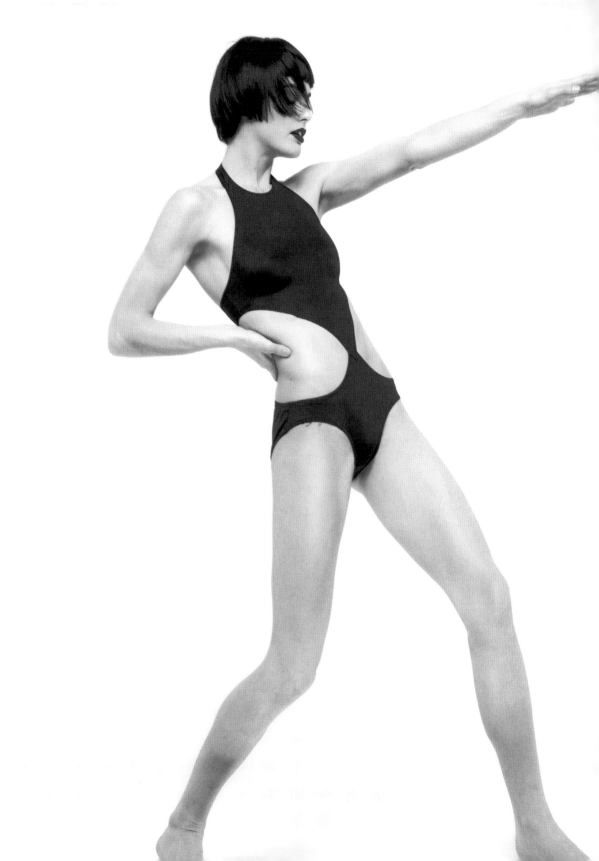

THINK ABOUT HOW YOU IDENTIFY YOURSELF THROUGH YOUR STYLE, BECAUSE THAT IS YOUR PERSONAL BRAND.

LET YOURS BE UNIQUELY YOU.

SHOES HELP DEFINE STYLE AND BODY LANGUAGE

CHOOSE SHOE STYLES THAT ARE APPEALING TO YOU PERSONALLY AND THAT YOU CAN WEAR COMFORTABLY SO YOUR BODY LANGUAGE WON'T BE COMPROMISED.

REPAIR SHOES...

BEFORE THEY ARE TOO
WORN-OUT SO THEY STAY IN
YOUR WARDROBE LONGER.
ESPECIALLY IF THEY ARE
YOUR FAVORITE PAIR.

SHOES CAN BE A PART OF YOUR COLLECTION FOR MANY, MANY YEARS.

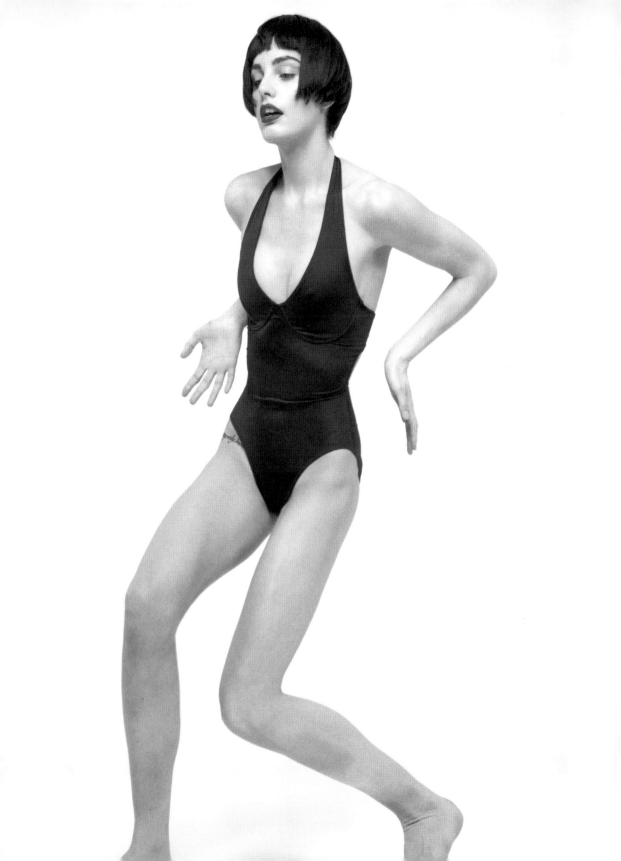

BUILD YOUR PERFECT WARDROBE AND DEVELOP YOUR PERSONAL STYLE

When I create a collection, I build outfits as part of the styling and merchandising of the line. A fashion tip we use at my design studio is to photograph the different looks to see what works best together. You can do the same every time you buy new styles, mixing them up to create as many looks as possible. Try on each outfit and be adventurous. Put things together you never considered before in order to find new ways to express yourself through your style and to make sure you really use every piece in your wardrobe. Don't forget to change shoes as you put together looks. The next time you need inspiration or have to dress for something unexpected, you won't have to shop because you will most likely have a look right in your closet. Keep editing over time to refine your assortment to a selection of clothing that gives you confidence. You'll know your statement style when you can look inside your closet and say, "That's it," because everything will be a favorite and will authentically express who you are.

TIPS ON SETTING UP YOUR CLOSET

An organized closet helps you edit what you really wear and what you don't need anymore. I like to set up our fashion closets at the office as well as my personal closet at home by color, then by fabric, and then by category: dresses, jumpsuits, tops, jackets, skirts, pants. It presents an orderly visual. All hangers should hook front-to-back in the same direction, and all clothing should face the same direction. Setting up dark to light is also easy on the eye. Next, a helpful strategy is to set up complete looks in a separate section at one end of your closet. You might want to consider, say, on a Sunday, arranging five outfits to wear Monday through Friday. Take the time to create fun looks that work for each day, with tops, bottoms, jackets, and accessories all together on one hanger. This saves me so much time throughout the week, especially when I am busy with day and evening commitments. I feel relaxed getting dressed, and I can spend more personal time each morning on meditation and preparing for the day. I do the same when I travel. I only bring the exact outfits for each day of the trip, not more. It is truly so efficient.

CLOTHES YOU LOVE AND
WEAR A LOT SHOULD BE DUPLICATED

This keeps favorite styles in good condition, and fresher longer. Once you know your style and the core of what works for you, especially if it is timeless, invest in duplicating some of those pieces.

• For me, bras are a no-brainer because a good bra that fits well improves the fit of all clothing. Spend time on this one.

• Find leggings you love, because if you feel good in them when you exercise, I think it boosts your workout . . . Crazy? No, true! And be sure they wash and wear well.

• I layer T-shirts in black jersey—long-sleeve, short-sleeve, tanks—and wear them with everything. I have six of each and rotate them in my wardrobe.

• For me, the Sleeping Bag Coat is an example of a great sustainable style that wears perfectly year after year. Having another one, exactly the same or in a print, breaks up the daily use in the winter and gives me variety for a style I love.

HOW TO PICK THE BEST SWIMSUIT FOR YOU!

THE BEST WAY TO CHOOSE SWIMWEAR IS TO:

• First, take off your clothes and stand in front of a mirror nude and assess your body. Your best assets are where you focus.

• Think of how the suit will look on you from every angle. After you analyze your body you can focus on the cuts that will complement your shape the most.

• I highly recommend shopping for suits online. Order from an assortment of brands, including your favorite. Order no fewer than four styles, maybe two sizes of the styles where you are unsure of the fit. Have them sent at the same time so you can try them all together. Use the mirror you trust and be sure you have access to daylight.

A LAST WORD ABOUT SWIMWEAR AND OBJECTIFICATION

I have designed swimwear for fifty years, and as a designer, I am pretty much known for it. During my Stop Objectification campaign, started in 2007, I was often confronted about the fact that I create some of the most provocative swim styles worn around the world. I was asked on occasion about the role fashion can play in objectifying women. If a woman feels powerful and confident about herself and her body, no swimsuit or piece of clothing is going to objectify her. I immediately thought of the members of the Olympic gold medal–winning U.S. women's volleyball team, who killed it in the tiniest little bikinis. Their bodies are part of their power. They were wearing the uniform of what they do. The furthest thing from anyone's mind was that they were being objectified. Every woman has the power to define how she wants to dress.

THINGS TO CONSIDER WHEN ORDERING:

1 ONE-PIECE, TWO-PIECE, AND BIKINI... TRY ALL THREE.
You might be surprised, but for sure you will establish a favorite.

2 IS THE SWIMSUIT FOR SWIMMING, SURFING, AND SPORTS?
Or is it for sitting by the pool, on a boat, or on the roof (using measures to monitor time and protection in the sun, I hope...)?

Once you define the purpose of the suit, the coverage, function, and style will be easier to determine.

3 BUST, WAIST, HIP... PROPORTION AND BALANCE.
Most swimwear is made with a standard set of proportions in mind, though very few people's bodies, not even most models', evenly match these measurements.

Determining the size and style that will flatter and fit most comfortably entails understanding your own proportions and which features you would like to accentuate. Try different styles and enjoy the adventure of finding a new silhouette.

4 NECKLINE, LEG LINE...
Try an assortment of necklines and leg openings to compare, and keep in mind how much support you want, or need, for your bust. A wide neckline tends to broaden the shoulders and a high leg line lengthens the leg. A long-line swimsuit extends the torso, and open backs add to the concept of a 360-degree view that keeps the eye moving around the body.

5 SOLIDS VERSUS PRINTS...
The theory has always been that solids are more flattering than prints, but this can work both ways. Trims and cutouts can also influence the look.

6 NEVER UNDERESTIMATE THE FUN ASPECT OF CLOTHING, ESPECIALLY SWIMWEAR.
If you feel good in it and it makes you happy, you will walk with just the right attitude to make it look great.

7 FINALLY, TAKE PICTURES OF YOURSELF IN EACH STYLE FROM THE FRONT, BACK, AND SIDE.
Review all photos and decide what to keep.

WHEN YOU TRAVEL, PACK LIGHT AND PACK SMART

MY YEARS AT NORTHWEST ORIENT AIRLINES INCLUDED TRAINING ON HOW TO PACK EFFICIENTLY. ONE OF THE KEY TIPS I LEARNED THEN AND STILL USE TODAY:

ROLL SMALL ITEMS AND KNITS AND PACK INSIDE A REUSABLE ZIPLOC BAG. ROLLING CLOTHES PREVENTS CREASES AND MAKES ROOM FOR SO MUCH MORE IN YOUR LUGGAGE. YOU CAN FIT A FEW ROLLS INTO A ONE-GALLON BAG. THEN, CLOTHES REQUIRING CLEANING CAN BE REROLLED BACK INTO THE ZIPLOC FOR THE RETURN HOME.

COUNT THE DAYS AND TIMES YOU WILL NEED A NEW OUTFIT. KEEP CLIMATE IN MIND AND THE VERSATILITY OF EACH STYLE YOU ARE PACKING.

WASH...
DON'T DRY-CLEAN

DRY CLEANING IS LIKE HAVING A PET THAT NEEDS MAINTENANCE WITHOUT THE UNCONDITIONAL LOVE. YOUR INVESTMENT IN CLOTHING THAT MUST BE DRY-CLEANED IS NEVER-ENDING. MANY OF THE CHEMICALS USED ARE NOT GOOD FOR THE ENVIRONMENT OR THE LONGEVITY OF YOUR CLOTHING. EVEN ECO-FRIENDLY DRY CLEANING IS NOT AS GOOD AS WASHING.

WORKLIFE

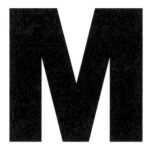**M**y mother's advice when I was eleven years old: "Be independent; learn how to earn your own way. Then you can choose someone you love versus someone to take care of you." I remember standing with my mother next to a washing machine she had received as a gift for Mother's Day as she told me this. It wasn't only the washing machine that inspired my mother's wise words, it was that her potential was so much greater, and she was realizing that she would not reach that potential in her lifetime. Her talents ran the gamut, from creativity to business. She was never at a loss for inspiration.

My mother was a very unique individual, definitely not like anyone else's mom. I am not sure she was the most maternal or nurturing type of mother, but she was artistic and adventurous. She was ahead of her time in every way, but was born to a generation where women weren't expected to be leaders. She was a leader in her approach to taking charge of her own life, though. She did everything from working in finance departments at various companies to creating the extraordinary window displays featuring the most elegant cakes at Schrafft's, a stylish eatery where ladies went in their hats and gloves for lunch and tea. She was ambitious, always working her way to management or as far as a woman could go.

MY MOTHER WAS AHEAD OF HER TIME IN EVERY WAY, BUT WAS BORN TO A GENERATION WHERE WOMEN WEREN'T EXPECTED TO BE LEADERS. SHE WAS A LEADER IN HER APPROACH TO TAKING CHARGE OF HER OWN LIFE, THOUGH.

She divorced my father at a time when people just didn't get divorced. This was an especially bold move if you were living in an Irish Catholic neighborhood and the church was a big part of the mindset of the community.

She remarried the only Jew in the neighborhood, the man who owned the candy store. Before we knew it, we were eating bagels, she was making gefilte fish, and we were driving to Miami every winter holiday. As a family, we adapted to another cultural mindset and belief system, and we did so seamlessly by her example.

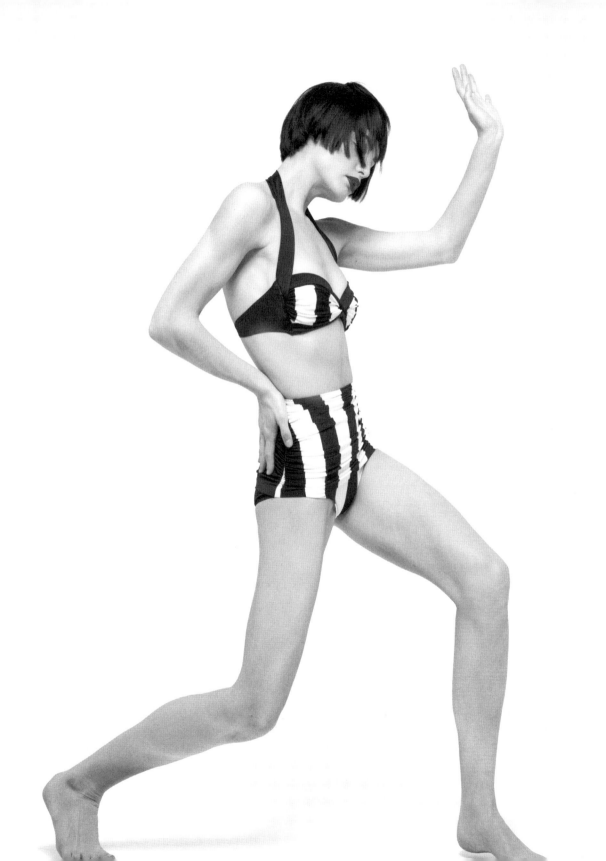

My mother literally transformed the candy store, which, in the fifties, was the center of everyone's universe. It was where the telephones and all of the magazines and newspapers were found. Many folks did not have a house phone, so this was where people came to make and receive calls.

My mother's transformation of the candy store was so successful that she and my stepfather soon expanded to an adjacent shop. She was a real partner and a driving force in all of the new additions that made the store about more than just candy.

I know that if she had been born at another time she could have run a company and been a business powerhouse. My mother's example was all I knew growing up. While I wasn't quite sure I fully understood her advice at the time it was given, I sure did later on.

I didn't start out thinking I would be an entrepreneur or a business owner, or even a fashion designer. I wanted to be a painter, so thinking about a career path wasn't my mindset, but it wasn't long before I understood that my art training was an amazing resource for living the creative life to which I aspired. Fashion and style in the 1960s were revolutionary and inventive, and I quickly found my medium. I immediately understood that I needed to find a way to combine art and commerce without relinquishing my dreams.

For me, starting a business in my early twenties meant I was driven by enthusiasm and vision, not experience or a formal business plan. I was so energized it gave me a false confidence I believed would steer me through the unknown. I found myself figuring it out along the way, and even now, every time I venture into a new project there is still some aspect of figuring it out as I go.

I learned to invest in my skills, gaining a firsthand understanding of what I didn't know, too, so I could push every aspect of my business forward and I didn't have to accept "no" for an answer. That was, and still is, the game-changer: When I was told something was impossible, I'd demonstrate how it was possible. For me, doing what has never been done is my talent, so I needed to have the ability to make that happen.

I am proud of being a self-taught woman in the business world. I still don't think of myself as being in a "career," but as more of an entrepreneur using my skills and passion to create as my labor of love. Maintaining my authenticity while staying in tune with the economy and business landscape so I can continue fifty years later is very satisfying.

When I initially went out on my own in 1976, men were extremely helpful, and both my lawyer and accountant, once I could afford them, provided fantastic advisory support. As I grew and developed licenses, all of my business was conducted with men. I understood my asset, which is my talent as a designer. Almost always I experienced respect and cooperation.

However, I had to work hard to prove myself for many years. For the most part and in general, a man who founded and ran a company and was also the designer would have been treated with more esteem. Once I felt confident about my worth as the president and business leader of the company, I was more forthcoming and vocal with my ideas and point of view. I learned how to frame my opinions and position in order to strategically achieve my goals.

Many of us, as women in any profession, have experienced frustration and routine humiliation during our career. On one occasion, after an intense negotiation in a conference room of all men, I made my case and actually won the argument politely. My opponent waited to leave behind me, and as we exited the room he patted me on the butt and said, "Good job!" I didn't say anything, even though I wanted to scream. I chose to let my accomplishment be the final word. This will not happen again, and today we have made great strides forward.

The most uplifting human opportunity is the ability to dream. Dreams are free of prejudice and life condition. No matter one's age or status, we can all dream. Men always have big dreams without consideration for the real possibility of the dream becoming real. Women have conventionally had more realistic dreams, but are now realizing that dreaming big can expand our potential. It is the dream that we have to visit and imagine when we are feeling hopeless and defeated by life's ups and downs. We need to dream, and we need to be lifted by the wonder of a dream coming true.

I spent my childhood dreaming. As I would sit quietly sketching, I would envision those dreams coming to life. I would walk around the city and imagine the world's possibilities and all that I would experience in New York and in the foreign countries I wished to one day visit. The wonderful thing about a dream is that it is limitless and it is free, and it can become the path to your purpose. **NK**

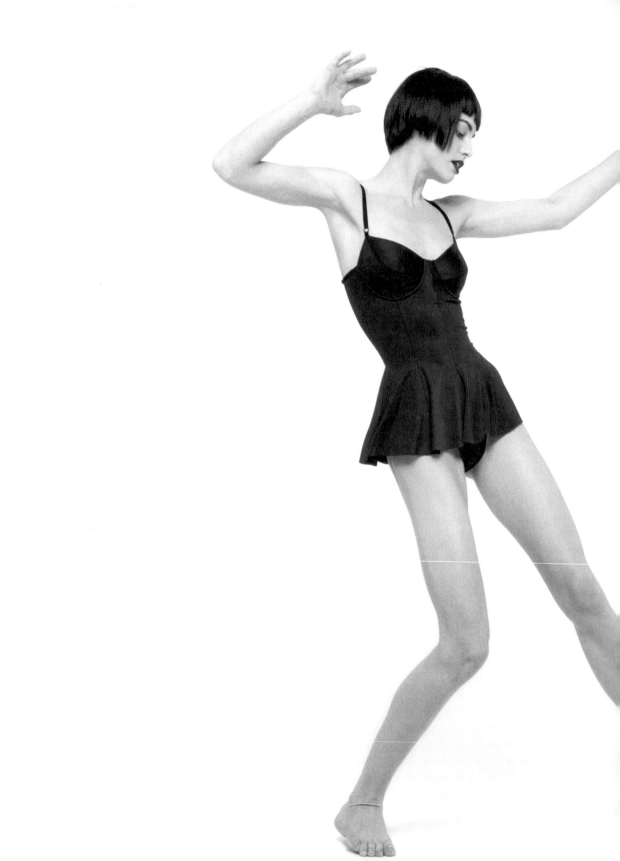

INVEST IN YOUR FUTURE, NOW!

EDUCATION, EXPERIENCE, COMMUNICATION, NETWORKING, AND PERSISTENT CURIOSITY WILL BE THE BEST INVESTMENT IN REACHING YOUR GOAL.

DO SOMETHING THAT SCARES YOU TO KEEP YOUR MIND SHARP.

THE WAY TO GROW IS TO PUSH THE BOUNDARIES IN AREAS YOU FIND CHALLENGING. THEN DOORS OPEN AND THE OPPORTUNITIES ARE EXCITING. IF IT FAILS OR THE RESULT OF YOUR ADVENTURE IS A NO!, MOVE ON, BUT BE SURE TO BE BOLD AND BRAVE AGAIN, LEARNING FROM THIS EXPERIENCE.

BE BOLD, BE BRAVE.

GIRLS COMPETE, WOMEN EMPOWER.

INSECURITY AND SELF-ESTEEM ISSUES CREATE FEAR. FEAR PRESENTS COMPETITION. HOWEVER, EXPERIENCE AND STRONG SELF-IMAGE BRING FORWARD GENEROSITY AND POWER.

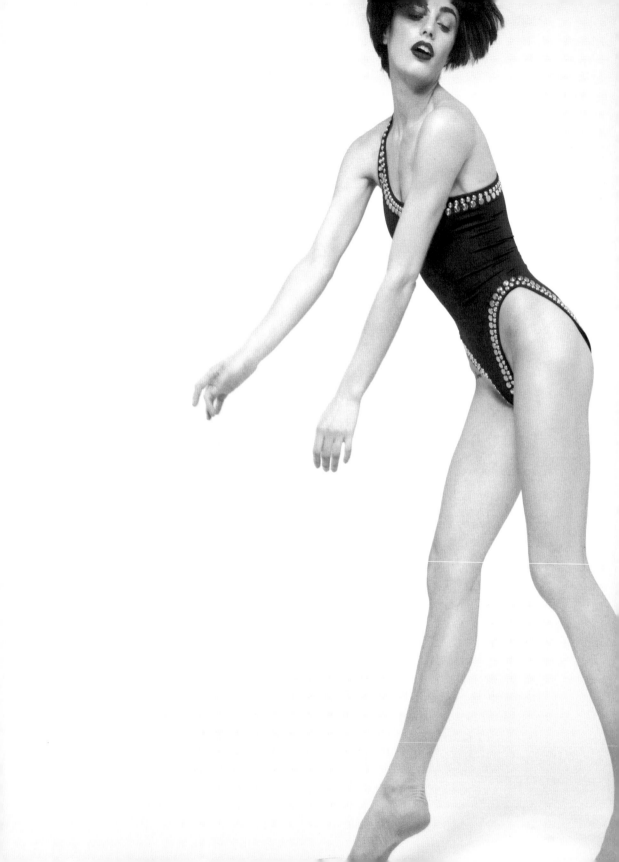

BE A GREAT EXAMPLE FOR ALL THE WOMEN AROUND YOU.

I THINK ABOUT ALL THE WOMEN WHO HAVE INSPIRED ME, AND HOW VALUABLE THEIR EXAMPLES HAVE BEEN IN HOW I MOVE THROUGH MY LIFE. IT IS IMPORTANT TO DO THE SAME FOR THE WOMEN FOLLOWING YOU.

IDEAS.

THE MORE IDEAS YOU HAVE,
THE MORE IDEAS YOU WILL HAVE.

MANY PEOPLE TREASURE AN

IDEA AND MAKE THAT THE IDEA

OF THEIR LIFETIME.

EXERCISE YOUR MIND, ESPECIALLY

THE IDEA PART OF YOUR BRAIN. EACH

NEW IDEA INSPIRES THE NEXT.

FOR EVERY TWENTY IDEAS YOU MIGHT HAVE, MAYBE ONE WILL HAVE THE POTENTIAL TO BECOME SUCCESSFUL.

IF YOU BELIEVE IN YOUR HEART THAT YOUR IDEAS HAVE VALUE AND YOU ARE WILLING TO GO ALL THE WAY TO MAKE THEM HAPPEN, THEY WILL.

PERSISTENCE AND PATIENCE ARE VIRTUES

A UNIQUE IDEA AND THE PASSION TO NAVIGATE THE TWISTS AND TURNS TO SEE IT THROUGH ARE THE SECRETS TO CONFIDENCE. THE INVESTMENT YOU MAKE SPIRITUALLY, EMOTIONALLY, AND PRACTICALLY IS NEEDED TO GET YOU THROUGH THE STAGES FROM PLAN TO REALIZATION.

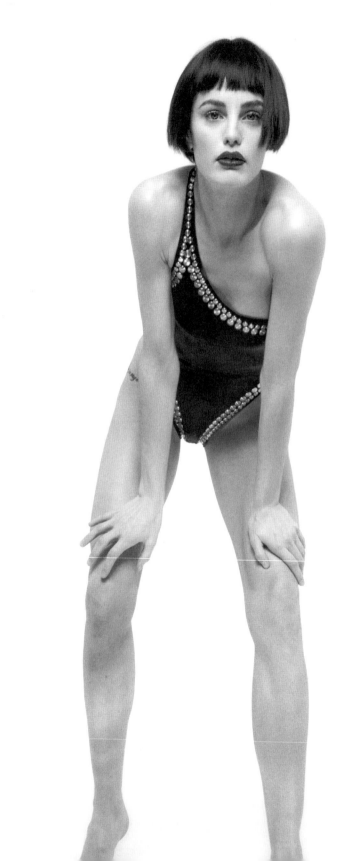

RESPECT IS LIKE MONEY:

YOU HAVE TO EARN IT.

RELATIONSHIPS ARE ETERNAL
IN BUSINESS AND IN LIFE

KEEP THIS IN MIND AND NURTURE THEM.
WHAT SEEMS LIKE A CONNECTION NO LONGER
RELEVANT IN YOUR LIFE CAN BECOME
IMPORTANT IN THE MOST UNEXPECTED WAY.

BE OPEN TO OPPORTUNITIES.

**MEET WITH ANYONE AND EVERYONE.
THERE IS ALWAYS SOMETHING TO LEARN
IN A MEETING, EVEN IF YOU SUSPECT
IT WILL NOT BE A FIT.**

THE MORE GLOBAL WE BECOME, THE SMALLER THE WORLD IS; THEREFORE YOU ARE SURE TO MEET AGAIN. BUSINESS ETIQUETTE IS A MUST.

EVERY INTERACTION IS IMPORTANT AND MUST BE TREATED RESPECTFULLY. EVEN THE DISAGREEMENTS NEED TO BE HANDLED PROFESSIONALLY. THIS IS YOUR REPUTATION.

BE AUTHENTIC, BE FAIR, AND DON'T SHUT THE DOOR ON REVISITING A RELATIONSHIP AT ANOTHER TIME OR ANOTHER PLACE, BECAUSE YOU MIGHT JUST WANT THAT TO HAPPEN IN A POSITIVE WAY DOWN THE ROAD, NO MATTER HOW UNLIKELY IT MAY SEEM AT THE TIME.

I STARTED IN BUSINESS IN 1967 AND HAD NO IDEA SO MANY RELATIONSHIPS WOULD COME AROUND FULL CIRCLE. WHEN GOODWILL EXISTS, IT IS QUITE EXTRAORDINARY.

DON'T BURN BRIDGES.

STORED ANGER MAKES US SICK.
IT TENDS TO BE HARD TO LET GO OF, AND,
MUCH WORSE, IT STARTS TO DEFINE A
PERSONALITY YOU DON'T WANT AS YOURS.

DON'T BE ANGRY WHEN THINGS GO WRONG IN BUSINESS.

ANGER CAN CERTAINLY BE A MOTIVATOR,
BUT IT IS DESTRUCTIVE, TOO. IF YOU'RE
NOT QUICK AT TURNING THAT ANGER
INTO PRODUCTIVE BEHAVIOR FOR CHANGE,
IT CAN TAKE YOU DOWN WITH IT.

**BE POSITIVE.
FIND AN UPSIDE AND A SOLUTION.**

FAILURE IS EMBARRASSING AND A REAL BLOW TO SELF-ESTEEM.

SMART ENTREPRENEURS WILL TELL YOU IT IS HOW YOU DEAL WITH YOUR FAILURES THAT SETS UP YOUR SUCCESSES.

ALLOW YOURSELF A LIMITED AMOUNT OF TIME TO RECOUNT THE EVENTS THAT LED TO FAILURE AND TO ASSESS THE DAMAGE. TAKE RESPONSIBILITY. LOOK AT OPTIONS FOR YOUR NEXT STEPS. GET ADVICE, THEN GET ON YOUR FEET AND KNOW YOU ARE NOT ALONE IN FAILURE.

JUST DON'T LET IT SHUT YOU DOWN.

REMEMBER: IN BUSINESS

"NO" IS ONLY A WORD...

IT CANNOT AND SHOULD NOT STOP YOU FROM TRYING TO PROMOTE YOUR IDEA AGAIN.

DETERMINATION IS NECESSARY
TO COPE WITH THE PERIODIC
CHALLENGES OF FAILURE.

AS WINSTON CHURCHILL SAID:

"SUCCESS IS THE ABILITY TO GO FROM ONE FAILURE TO ANOTHER WITH NO LOSS OF ENTHUSIASM."

WHEN YOU BELIEVE IN WHAT YOU ARE DOING,
YOU NEVER LOSE ENTHUSIASM.

MY ATTITUDE IS BASED ON
THE CONFIDENCE I HAVE
DEVELOPED THAT IF ONE IDEA
FAILS, I CAN COME UP WITH
ANOTHER, BECAUSE THAT IS
WHAT I LOVE TO DO.

ENTREPRENEURSHIP
IS AN ATTITUDE
TOWARD HOW YOU
ACHIEVE YOUR
CAREER GOALS.

APPROACHING EVERYTHING YOU DO AS AN ENTREPRENEUR MEANS YOU ARE WILLING TO TAKE FULL RESPONSIBILITY FOR EVERY ACTION AND DECISION TO MAKE IT A SUCCESS.

THE ALTERNATIVE IS LOOKING AT EVERYTHING AS AN EMPLOYEE. THIS PERSON RARELY IMAGINES A LEADERSHIP POSITION.

IT IS ALL ABOUT CHOICE.

FROM THE BEGINNING OF MY CAREER, I DECIDED
WHAT I WANTED WAS TO HAVE TOTAL FREEDOM
TO BE CREATIVE EVERY DAY OF MY LIFE.

BE OPEN AND FLEXIBLE IN YOUR THINKING WHILE MAINTAINING THE INTEGRITY OF YOUR GOALS.

IN ORDER TO DO SO, I NEEDED TO WEIGH THE
OPTIONS FOR MY BUSINESS. I COULD HAVE PARTNERS,
I COULD GET BOUGHT OUT, OR I COULD WORK FOR
OTHER COMPANIES. I CHOSE THE MOST APPEALING
AND PROBABLY THE LEAST LUCRATIVE AVENUE:

THE RESULT OF THE ENTREPRENEURIAL
APPROACH IS THAT I AM LIVING A CREATIVE LIFE
AND I STILL OWN MY COMPANY AND MY NAME.

WHEN YOU ARE THE HEAD OF A BUSINESS, YOUR MOOD, YOUR ATTITUDE, AND YOUR PERSONALITY BECOME THE TEMPERAMENT OF THE COMPANY.

A STRONG SENSE OF CONFIDENCE AND A PROFOUND SENSE OF HUMOR MAKE SUCCESS MORE LIKELY.

IT TOOK ME YEARS TO TRULY UNDERSTAND WHAT THAT MEANT. AS SOON AS I DID, I REALIZED PEOPLE WANT STRENGTH IN THEIR LEADERS. IT MAKES EVERYONE FEEL SECURE AND STABLE. NOT EVERY DAY WILL BE PERFECT, BUT INSTEAD OF RESPONDING WITH ANGER WHEN A DIFFICULT SITUATION PRESENTS ITSELF, HUMOR, IF YOU CAN MANAGE IT, IS ALWAYS A BETTER APPROACH.

COMMUNICATION.

EMAILS ARE A GREAT WAY TO DOCUMENT CONVERSATIONS AND COMMITMENTS. FACE-TO-FACE MEETINGS ARE IMPORTANT, AS WELL, TO INTERACT ON A PERSONAL LEVEL AND DEVELOP A BOND. AND IF YOU CAN'T MEET, VIDEO CONFERENCE IS SUPER HELPFUL, ESPECIALLY FOR LONG-DISTANCE MEETINGS.

GO OUT OF YOUR WAY TO MAKE CONNECTIONS HAPPEN.

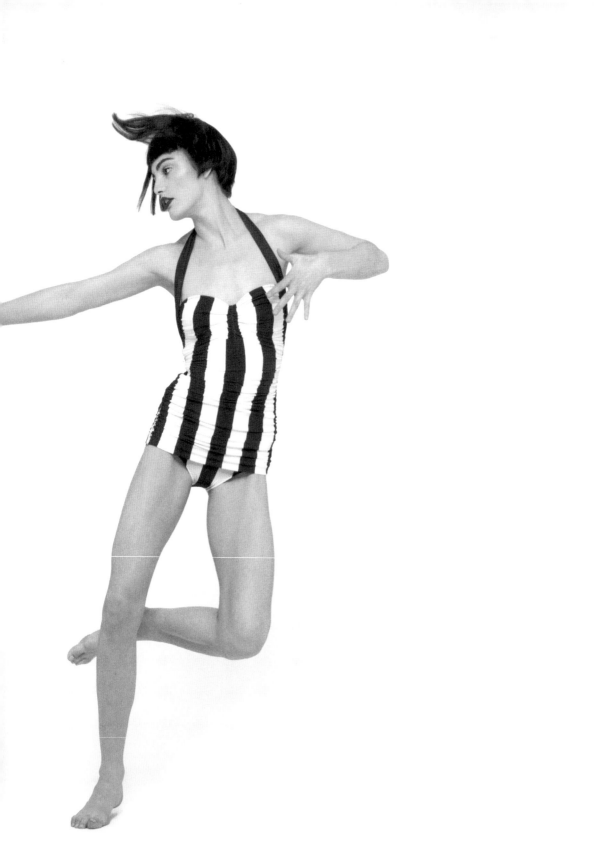

DO IT FOR JOY... AND YOU CAN DO IT FOREVER!

GETTING

INTERNSHIPS.

While deciding your career path, internships can be extremely beneficial. Pick a brand, a company, or a project that interests you. Interview with the company, offer hard work, and demonstrate your openness to participate as a fast learner. While you are there, study the behavior of the successful people and the best practices in the workplace. Offer to help anyone who looks like they could use your assistance, while being sure to successfully complete the assignments you are given each day. This experience will make you more valuable and will also provide an inside look into that particular world. This is great advice for graduates straight out of school, or anyone looking to make a change. I have a friend who, after being quite successful in the financial world, concluded he wanted to do something different. He made good money, saved it, and decided he wanted to create something. He wanted to build low-income housing in a special way. He interviewed for an internship in his forties and got it. He asked for no salary and worked hard and contributed to the company as he learned about the industry he was determined to make his next venture. This may not be for everyone, but it can be a valuable option for some people.

STARTED

MENTORS. GET ONE.

Have mentors and business professionals to use as your sounding board. They will be helpful in giving you direction and feedback, which in turn will inform how you make the ultimate decisions. Ask for help. Contact people you admire and tell them what you do and ask for advice. It will be a rare instance that someone doesn't help you if you ask. The bigger they are, the more generous the response will be. I remember contacting the woman who ran Henri Bendel in the seventies. I thought she was so smart and innovative in her approach to retail. The store was a magical place. She was responsible for all of the talent hired to make it happen. I just called the store and asked if I could speak with her. I explained to her assistant the reason I wanted to meet her. I got a call back the same week and met with her soon after. Seeing her office, observing her body language, and receiving her recommendations had an incredible impact on decisions I made going forward. Take the chance and contact your inspirational person and see what happens.

BE WILLING TO SHIFT GEARS.

By doing so, you will have better results in the end. Setting goals and crafting a plan with steps to make your project come alive is the starting point. However, in business everyone knows circumstances sometimes suggest other avenues in order to reach your goals. If you are flexible and open to change, the outcome might in fact turn out better than what you originally planned. I studied painting and life drawing and felt convinced it was my calling. And I was quite good at it. Practical adjustments were made in order for me to find a way to pay rent and to be self-sufficient. After studying fashion illustration, once I graduated from school I decided it was time to see the world. It was during my weekend trips to London during the 1960s while working for Northwest Orient Airlines that I truly understood how perfectly fit I was for fashion and the extraordinarily creative time in which I was living. I traveled the road and kept my mind open to new opportunities. It happened organically, and perhaps that's the way the Universe plans it.

SET YOURSELF UP FOR SUCCESS

WHEN STARTING A NEW BUSINESS, ALWAYS ESTIMATE THAT YOU WILL SPEND MORE TIME THAN YOU COULD EVER IMAGINE ON MAKING IT HAPPEN.

Anything new means just that . . . It is new. Therefore, no matter how well you plan and how much advice you get, there will be some aspect of it that may surprise you. The fact that you need to invest more time and probably more money than you expected seems inevitable, so count on it and put it into your plan.

AN ENTREPRENEUR IS INHERENTLY AN INNOVATOR AND MUST BE CAPABLE OF THINKING IN UNCONVENTIONAL WAYS.

I liken this to cooking with a recipe and then you realize you are out of two of the ingredients. You want to save the meal, and to do so you have to be creative. It is through this mindset and practical approach to success that you will discover the ability to quickly pivot and adapt.

SALESMANSHIP

You must sell your idea if you want to succeed. Storytelling and connecting directly to an audience of like-minded people is the only way to create an action or reaction. Salesmanship is a skill, an actual art form when done well. You must believe deeply in your narrative to be effective. I was incredibly shy, but my survival as a designer meant I needed to speak up to tell my story. Many creative people feel uncomfortable selling their work themselves. Selling is not successful if that is all you are doing. Telling your story honestly and openly, communicating your dream and the joy of your creative abilities, is the best selling approach. This is true for anyone who has a dream project and wants it to become a thriving business.

TIME MANAGEMENT...

...means working to the max with a plan in the period of time delegated for work. Distractions like texting and social media will cause longer workdays and less time to develop a balanced life. If you are a structured person and do well with this at work, then I say apply structure to scheduling personal time in your calendar, too—then it is clear you are booked, taking care of you.

TAKE GOOD CARE OF YOURSELF AND OTHERS

SUPPORT WOMEN, EDUCATE MEN.

Experienced women must be kind and generous to young women starting out. Remember that you, too, were insecure when you were in your twenties. Be a mentor to someone who will then become a mentor, who will then become a mentor, and the chain goes on. The more we bring men into our lives, the better the communication and the better their understanding and behavior will be. Educating men is best achieved by example. We can share stories about good examples of support, and stories about painful experiences of inappropriate behavior. No father will ever want his daughter to be objectified; he will be the best advocate for women once he is informed and aware. Mothers need new tools to encourage their sons to cultivate admiration and respect for women. We must encourage men to get in touch with their feminine side in the way we are learning that we are comfortable with our masculine side.

COMMUNITY.

From the earliest phase of your career, be sure to find a
way to be of service to the community. Find compatible
organizations to support and commit to a cause or
movement that enhances the lives of others. This helps keep
perspective on values and brings balance to your life.
Since the late eighties, I have been involved with New York
City's public schools. I have mentored fashion classes, offered
internships, and provided support to help the students.
The by-product of this relationship with my company alone
is that it makes us feel good. We are energized, and it is
a source of positive reinforcement. To create the ultimate
positive energy, keep your cup half-full by giving.

STOP OBJECTIFICATION.

Throughout this book I have written about my experiences with objectification,
as a young woman applying for my first job and even as the head of my own
company. Objectification in the workplace is disappearing, but it does still exist.
Objectification takes such a toll on our self-esteem that we very often keep the
incidents to ourselves. The accumulation of secrets erodes our confidence
and undermines our ability to reach our potential. By sharing our painful stories,
we bring awareness to these issues and we inspire other women to free themselves of the secrets they hide of these occurrences. Share your personal
stories and get support for how to handle situations as they arise. Be open and
communicate concerns to those involved and to others, so that issues are
defused immediately.

AUTHENTIC
BEAUTY

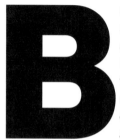**B**eauty is at its best when it is authentic. The true essence of beauty is that we are all unique. Don't try to be someone else's beautiful; be the most beautiful you! My personal experiences with self-esteem are no different from other women's. I grew up in an Irish Catholic neighborhood with the most beautiful children. They either had curly blond hair and big blue eyes or red hair and green eyes or dark hair with pale freckled skin. I had brown hair and olive skin, and my nose didn't turn up, it just kept growing. I certainly questioned my look, and often felt like an ugly duckling because I was different. Beauty, to me, was defined by their terms and coloring.

As a teenager, I decided that since I was not pretty, I would come up with unique looks that were of my making. I created hair and makeup styles influenced by the elite fashion magazines of the time: teased hair, individual lashes, strong Jean Shrimpton eyeliner, and pale lips. Most sixteen-year-olds were not following the fashion magazines; they were finding influence in the more plentiful celebrity magazines that featured styled portraits of Sophia Loren, Marilyn Monroe, and for teens, Sandra Dee and Ricky Nelson. Yup, I'm dating myself here big-time.

I put every ounce of artistry I had into my hair and makeup—which took an hour and a half to do—as an almost daily creative project. I would wear clothes that differentiated me even further from my peers, so I couldn't be judged by the prevailing standards. *Hello!* I found my talent and my own style, but I still never personally identified as beautiful.

BEAUTY IS VERY MUCH ABOUT DEVELOPING PERSONAL STYLE: A SIGNATURE THAT GIVES YOU CONFIDENCE AND REFLECTS YOUR IDENTITY. IT EVOLVES THROUGH TIME AS YOU MATURE AND EXPERIENCE LIFE.

The beauty and fashion industries have perpetuated myths of ideal beauty, convincing us that beauty is not who we are as individuals, but what we should aspire to look like. The products women are convinced they need in order to be good enough, pretty enough, and young enough are the very things

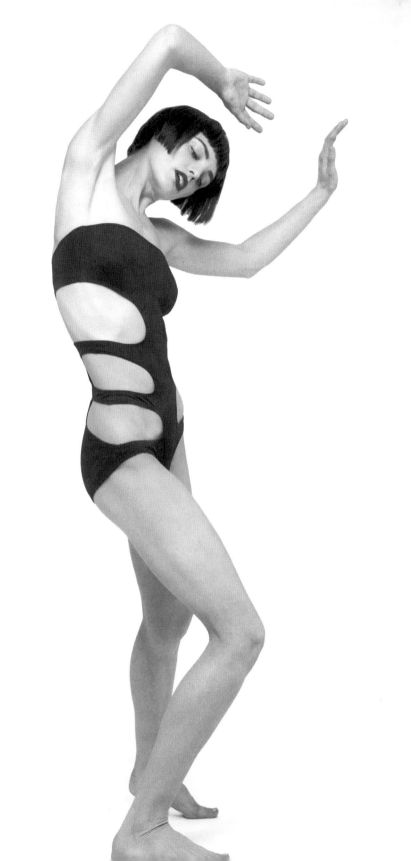

that often make us feel inadequate. Self-esteem is everything when it comes to reaching our potential. Having it undermined by advertisements of false promises impacts a woman's self-worth from an early age.

Today, an appreciation of the authentic self is inspiring more and more women to embrace their own singularity. No one else has what you have, and *that is your power*.

Similar to fashion, beauty is very much about developing personal style: a signature that gives you confidence and reflects your identity. It evolves through time as you mature and experience life.

Each of us makes a choice about how we enhance our individuality. You are saying so much about who you are by how you wear your hair and makeup. It is certainly a valid opportunity to create the image you want to project; however, there are alternate beauty choices, as well. I always feel that a smiling face with a twinkle in the eye tells such a great story about the people we meet. For me, this is the image that forms the first impression. Makeup either adds to or complicates that story.

It took me time to appreciate the difference. I wore makeup throughout my twenties and thirties. I didn't have a clear sense of who I was yet. I loved doing my makeup. I felt like I was playing a role in the different looks I wore. I hid behind my makeup mastery. This was my pretend self. My hair and clothing matched the fun fantasy of that period of my life.

At a certain point, I realized that the more empowered I felt as I gained experience through life, the more I wanted to show my true self. How much makeup do you need if you are living a healthy lifestyle? Most probably, there is very little to cover up. The older I got, the more I realized my skin looks so much better when it glows naturally. I felt confident enough to go make-up-free if I wanted.

Today, my beauty style is based upon taking care of my skin. I have been following the same routine since 1993, when I decided to stop wearing foundation. When I met Horst Rechelbacher, the genius behind Aveda and an outspoken pioneer of the natural and clean beauty movement, he shared his knowledge about the suspicious ingredients in many cosmetics and brought my attention to issues within the beauty industry. Working with chemists, I developed a skin-care concept using safe ingredients that cleanse, exfoliate, moisturize, and create a glow. Since I decided to go bare and stick to an easy plan, I feel good about my skin.

Ever since Horst's reality check about the amount of lipstick women may inadvertently consume each year, simply by applying it, and its potential impact on health, I've stopped wearing my trademark red lips. I learned that nail polish was no better, so I have bare nails now, too. I accent my eyebrows and lashes, dab on some lip stain, and I feel: That's me. My ethnicity presents dark shadows under my eyes, so I use dots of highlighter as a brightener. This simple solution works best when I am eating properly, sleeping well, and working out.

AUTHENTICITY ENHANCED IS MY BEAUTY PREFERENCE, SINCE BEING ME IS DEFINITELY EASIER THAN TRYING TO LOOK LIKE SOMEONE ELSE.

All in all, I approach my personal care as easy care, same as my collection and my personal style: timeless and comfortable but fun and expressive at the same time.

I only started to wear glasses at fifty, so I designed eyewear that is flattering for most face shapes, and I have been wearing the cat-eye tortoise frames for some time. I added tinted lenses so I can use them both at my computer and outdoors. My blunt-cut bangs, which have become a trademark over time, work well with my square face. Instead of trying to nuance the shape, I am going with it! I rinse my hair every day after working out, so it needs to be a style that is easy to maintain and as close to my natural texture as possible. My hair is straight, but frizzy at the same time. I used to have it flat-ironed, but after so much breakage week after week, I gave it up, and now that it is healthy, I am letting it grow naturally. After a lot of research, I finally created a three-in-one shampoo, conditioner, and styler that tames the frizzies and keeps my hair shiny and smooth. Now I am free to take a shower, smooth in some product, and be on my way.

Authenticity enhanced is my beauty preference, since being me is definitely easier than trying to look like someone else.

My question is, what works for you? What reflects your sensibility and treats each of your features as a best asset? Natural skin, groomed brows, a swipe of mascara, and bangs I trim myself is my preference. Have you found yours? NK

SMILING...

...IS A BEAUTY TIP!

USE IT AS OFTEN AS POSSIBLE THROUGHOUT THE DAY. IT IS FRIENDLY AND WELCOMING, AND EVERYONE LOOKS BETTER WITH A SMILE.

TAKE PRIDE IN YOUR INDIVIDUALITY.

THIS IS WHAT MAKES YOU UNIQUE AND INTERESTING. MY SIXTH-GRADE TEACHER WROTE IN MY GRADUATION ALBUM, "KNOW THYSELF."

EACH OF US HAS A STORY.

BEING THE AUTHOR OF YOUR OWN LIFE IS FAR MORE INTERESTING THAN IMITATING ANOTHER'S LIFE.

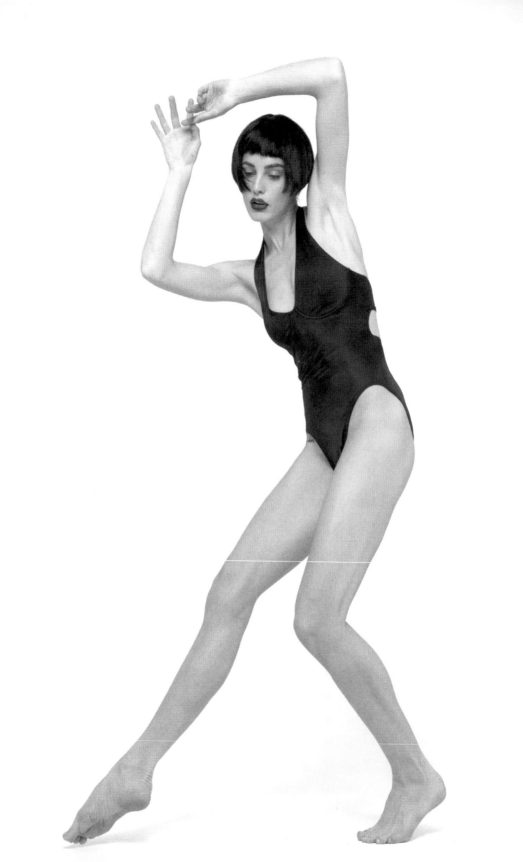

WE ARE AT OUR MOST BEAUTIFUL WHEN WE ARE OUR AUTHENTIC SELVES.

ENHANCE YOUR NATURAL LOOK BY PROMOTING HEALTHY SKIN SO THE MAKEUP YOU WEAR IS FOR DEFINITION, NOT TO HIDE OR DISGUISE THE REAL YOU.

I HAD A LONG LOOK AT MY MOTHER'S GORGEOUS SKIN AND UNDERSTOOD THERE WAS A GENETIC FACTOR AT PLAY, BUT THERE WERE LIFESTYLE CHOICES THAT ADDED TO HER BEAUTY, TOO. SHE WAS JUICING AND WORKING OUT TO JACK LALANNE, THE FITNESS GURU OF THE SIXTIES, AND TAKING SUPPLEMENTS ALL THROUGH MY CHILDHOOD. THE FACT THAT SHE DIDN'T SIT IN THE SUN, EVER, ACCOUNTED FOR HER CLEAR, MILKY COMPLEXION, FREE OF FRECKLES AND SUNSPOTS EVEN INTO HER EIGHTIES. SHE NEVER USED SOAP ON HER FACE; SHE WOULD USE POND'S COLD CREAM TO WIPE OFF HER MAKEUP AND MOISTURIZE. SHE USED A WARM WASHCLOTH, AND THAT WAS IT.

LOOK AT YOUR MOTHER'S SKIN, HAIR, HANDS, AND BODY TYPE.

CHANCES ARE YOU WILL LOOK VERY MUCH THE SAME AS YOU GET OLDER. DECIDE WHAT THE BENEFITS ARE OF YOUR GENETIC POOL, THEN ACT ACCORDINGLY.

WHILE I TAKE AFTER MY FATHER'S BASQUE COLORING, I APPRECIATE MY GENETIC POOL, AND I KNOW I MUST DO ALL I CAN TO ADAPT MY LIFESTYLE TO PROTECT MY SKIN.

YOU SEE SWEAT, I SEE A GLOW!

SWEAT FOR GLOWING SKIN AND TO RELEASE TOXINS.

THE LUMINOUS SKIN OF SOMEONE WHO WAS JUST WORKING OUT IS A HEALTHY LOOK. BLOOD IS FLOWING; SKIN LOOKS DEWY AND ALIVE.

LET YOUR SKIN BREATHE. A FOUNDATION-FREE FACE IS LIBERATING!

ADD A HEALTHY DIET, REGULAR EXERCISE, AND A GOOD NIGHT'S SLEEP FOR THE BEST RECIPE FOR A RADIANT COMPLEXION.

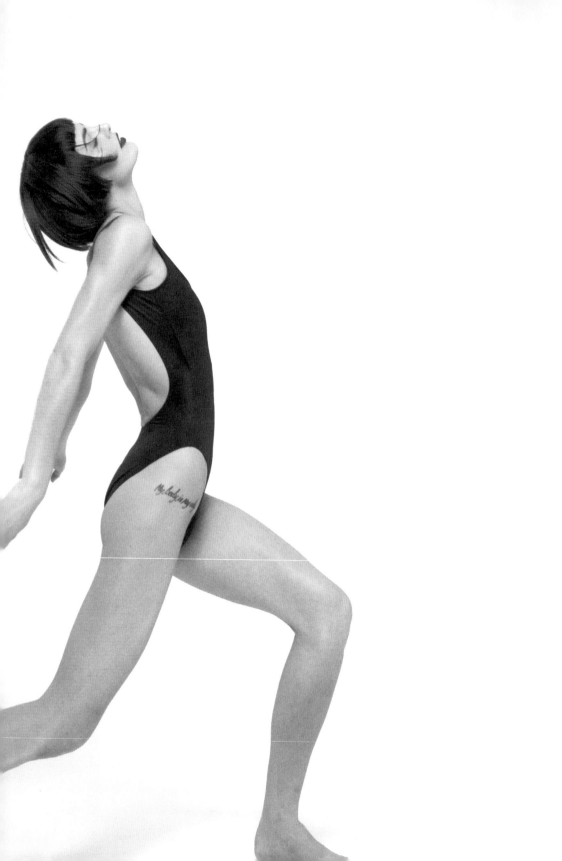

EYEBROWS...

... ARE THE ACCENT TO YOUR FACE.

BE CAREFUL NOT TO OVERGROOM... ... AND CHANGE YOUR NATURAL EXPRESSION.

MOST NAIL POLISHES AND MATERIALS USED
IN MANICURES ARE CHEMICALS. EITHER
FIND SAFE POLISH, OR USE NONE AT ALL.
TRY CULTIVATING HEALTHY, STRONG NAILS . . .
. . . IF YOUR NAILS ARE HEALTHY YOU WON'T
NEED TO COVER THEM.

NATURAL, UNPAINTED MANICURES ARE HEALTHY AND MAINTAIN A TIMELESS LOOK.

TO SOFTEN CUTICLES, SOAK NAILS IN WARM
OLIVE OIL FOR FIVE MINUTES.

FACIALS ARE HELPFUL FOR STIMULATING THE SKIN.

THERE ARE MANY TYPES OF FACIALS THAT CAN HAVE AN IMPACT ON SKIN'S TONE AND TEXTURE.

WHETHER AT HOME OR AT A FACIALIST, THIS IS A SKIN MAINTENANCE PLAN THAT SHOULD BE AS IMPORTANT AND AS SIMPLE AS OTHER SELF-CARE PRACTICES.

BE SURE WHEREVER YOU GO THAT PRODUCTS FORMULATED WITH NATURAL AND CLEAN INGREDIENTS ARE USED.

SHINY, HEALTHY HAIR LOOKS GOOD IN ANY STYLE.

EACH OF US HAS

A DIFFERENT

RELATIONSHIP WITH

OUR HAIR.

I HAVE FOUND THAT WORKING WITH THE NATURAL LOOK OF MY HAIR, THROUGH A GREAT CUT AND THE RIGHT PRODUCTS, TAKES THE LEAST EFFORT AND GIVES ME THE MOST FREEDOM.

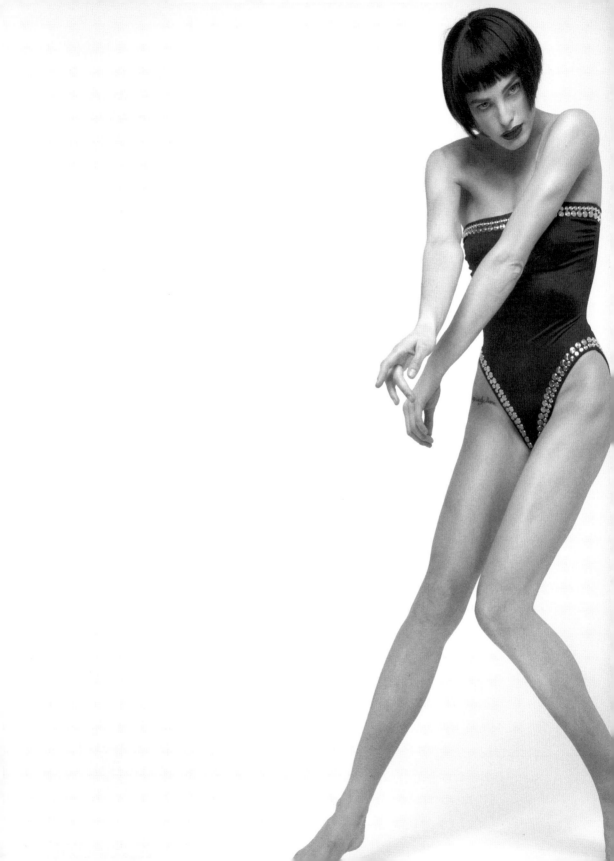

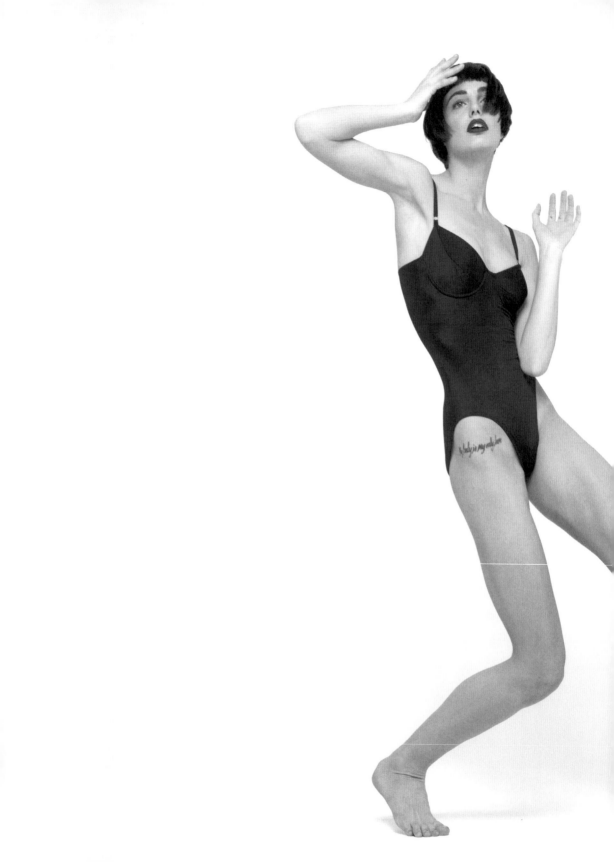

LIPSTICK...

...IS BELIEVED TO BE INADVERTENTLY INGESTED IN POUNDS BY WOMEN OVER THE COURSE OF THEIR LIFETIMES. RETHINK WHAT YOU PUT ON YOUR LIPS.

PLANT-BASED LIP COLORS AS WELL AS FOOD-BASED STAINS ARE PRETTY AND A HEALTHY ALTERNATIVE. BEET JUICE AND COCONUT OIL MAKE A GREAT DEEP LIP STAIN.

THERE ARE SO MANY AFFORDABLE
COSMETIC TECHNIQUES THAT CAN
CHANGE A PERSON'S LIFE AND RESULT
IN BETTER SELF-ESTEEM. WHATEVER
YOU DECIDE, KEEP THE BEST VERSION
OF YOURSELF IN MIND.

THERE IS NOTHING WRONG WITH COSMETIC ENHANCEMENTS...

...AS LONG AS YOU ARE ENHANCING AND NOT
GOING INTO THE WITNESS PROTECTION PROGRAM.

MAKE SURE DIET AND EXERCISE ARE PART
OF THE PLAN FOR ACHIEVING YOUR BEST LOOK,
BECAUSE THESE YOU CAN CONTROL.

TRY AN ACUPUNCTURE FACIAL FOR A REFRESHED LOOK.

WHEN ACUPUNCTURE IS FOCUSED ON THE FACE, THE RESULT IS GLOWING SKIN AND A RENEWED SPARKLE IN THE EYES. IT'S A HOLISTIC EXPERIENCE THAT RESTORES BOTH MIND AND BODY.

WHEN I DO IT ON A REGULAR BASIS — ONCE A WEEK, ONCE A MONTH — I FIND THE CUMULATIVE EFFECT TO BE VERY POSITIVE. I REALLY DO SEE A DIFFERENCE. I DON'T JUST FEEL GOOD; I FEEL GOOD ABOUT MYSELF.

GROOM YOURSELF CONFIDENTLY.

BE YOUR AUTHENTIC SELF. TRY ANYTHING THAT FEELS RIGHT FOR YOU.

A REALLY GOOD TIP IS TO TAKE A PHOTO IN AN ELEVATOR OR BATHROOM WITH FLUORESCENT LIGHTING AND ALSO OUTDOORS ON A SUNNY DAY. IF YOU LIKE WHAT YOU SEE, THEN IT IS WORKING.

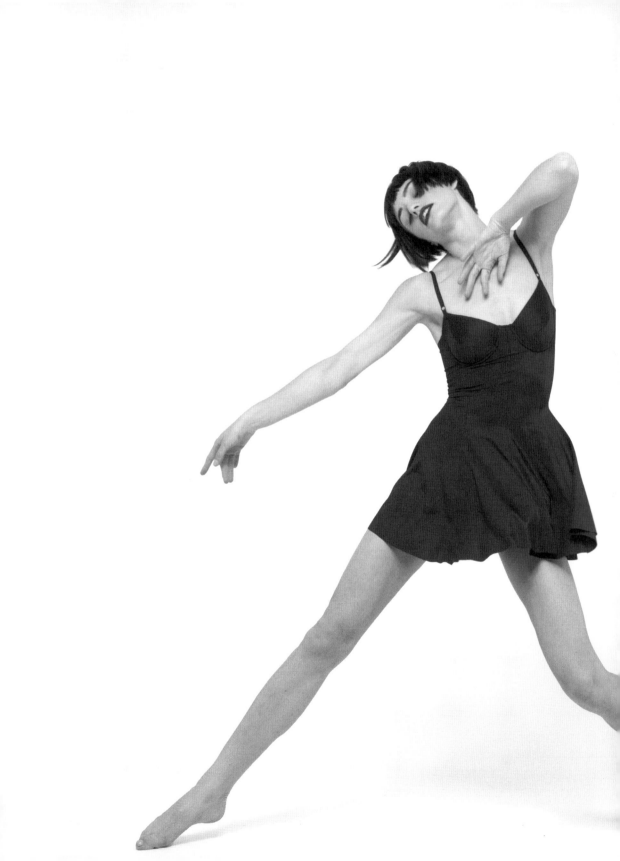

KNOW WHAT'S INSIDE YOUR PRODUCTS

THE WORD "CLEAN" IN PERSONAL CARE AND BEAUTY REFERS TO THE IMPORTANCE OF INGREDIENT SAFETY.

My awareness about cosmetic ingredients began seriously when I opened the Wellness Café after 9/11. I wanted alternative self-care formulations that would support the immune system. The more I learned, the more I realized how vulnerable we are when we aren't educated about what is in the products we use. I thought I was very informed until I recently upgraded the SKINLINE for NORMALIFE. I sourced timeless, proven ingredients, focusing on natural and organic, and worked with chemists who follow the most stringent protocols. In Manchester, England, where I went especially to discuss ingredient safety, the chemists were kind enough to tolerate my persistent questions. I learned that sometimes man-made ingredients are safer and more effective in a formula than some natural raw materials. What happens when you blend certain ingredients together can create something wonderful, or maybe not. Sometimes, the best formulations are a combination of non-toxic synthetic and natural ingredients. Make sure you are aware of what is in the products you use and the food you eat.

USE ALOE TO PURIFY, HEAL, AND HYDRATE

Use aloe as a **hair conditioner**.

Look for moisturizers containing natural aloe vera for **face and body**.

Mix aloe juice with other liquids, like coconut water, to use as a **digestive aid**.

Apply fresh aloe gel directly from the leaves of the plant to **calm irritated skin or sunburn**.

A TIMELESS, ALL-NATURAL SCRUB IS GREAT FOR STIMULATING THE SKIN

In ancient times, Cleopatra exfoliated with olive oil and sand.

Olive oil has numerous skin benefits, from anti-inflammatory properties to its wealth of the antioxidant squalane. Mineral-rich **sea salt** is naturally detoxifying, softening, and helps restore pH balance.

Try a gentle, hydrating extra virgin olive oil and sea salt **facial scrub**.

A sea salt **bath** soothes muscles and relaxes both body and mind.

GREEN TEA MASKS ARE A PERFECT ANTIOXIDANT FOR THE SKIN

I DRINK A CUP OR TWO OF GREEN TEA EVERY DAY. THE POLYPHENOLS IT CONTAINS ARE AN INCREDIBLE SOURCE OF ANTIOXIDANTS, WHICH HAVE BEEN SHOWN TO HAVE BENEFITS FOR THE SKIN WHEN APPLIED TOPICALLY, TOO.

GREEN TEA CAN HELP CALM REDNESS AND INFLAMMATION AND PROTECT SKIN FROM FREE RADICAL DAMAGE. THE SMALL AMOUNT OF CAFFEINE IT CONTAINS ALSO HELPS ALLEVIATE PUFFINESS AROUND THE EYES.

This DIY mask is easy to do:

1 Place a paper towel on a dinner plate.

2 Pour a small amount of freshly brewed cool or room-temperature green tea on the paper towel.

3 Drain any excess liquid.

4 Lie back with your head on a towel and place the paper towel over your face.

5 Relax and breathe in a meditative manner.

6 Remove the towel when you are ready, and pat dry.

DO FACIAL EXERCISES FOR A FIT FACE

JUST LIKE PHYSICAL FITNESS, FACE FITNESS INCREASES BLOOD FLOW, FIRMNESS, AND MUSCLE TONE

My mother did a series of facial exercises that were similar to an active facial. She would do exaggerated facial movements such as a puckered *oooohhhhh* and a wide-mouthed *aaaaaahhhhhh*. She massaged her face in circular movements at her temples and upward strokes with her fingers under her cheekbones. I recently had a facial, and the facialist presented herself as my "face trainer" and literally reenacted all of my mother's timeless facial exercises.

ON
PURPOSE

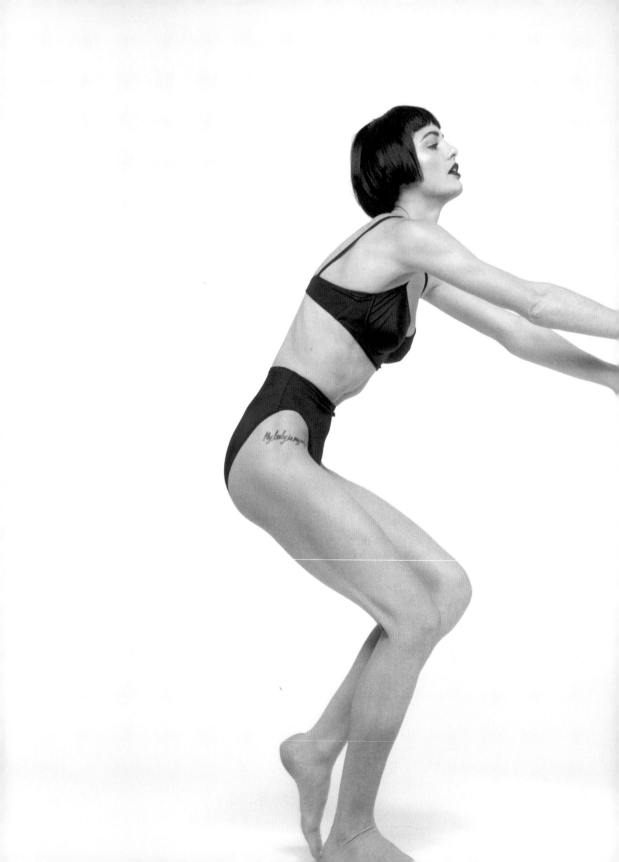

The minute you reflect upon what your purpose is in this lifetime, you can commit to it, and the easier it will be to maintain focus and stay on course. Ambling from day to day, feeling disappointed that your dreams aren't being fulfilled, is the alternative. Purpose is everything. It is why we are here. It is what gives our lives meaning. Knowing your purpose and acting on it to the last breath of your life is so important for each and every one of us. If we have a positive mission for our lifetime, then we live each day in a way that creates results.

I have thought long and hard about my purpose for the last forty years, and even more so recently. I am now able to recognize how I can manifest it to help my soul evolve and to try to help others, which I believe we all need to do.

I intuitively understood over time that my purpose was even more meaningful than my dream of living a creative life. I realized that I could use my abilities to be of service to women by helping them feel good about themselves, because this is what I have been doing for myself over the years, and I could make it real for others.

Clothes are a powerful tool for identifying who we are and the roles we play at different times in our lives. They can empower; they can help us have fun, or simply express our personal style, attitude, and outlook. Clothing is so personal, and the connection to a brand can be very intimate because, as designers, we wrap our styles around you, and it is like a big hug.

Over five decades, I have listened to women as they have told me stories about how they felt in my clothing. I am sure other designers have similar experiences. I have met women who have married in my clothing, met their partners and marked milestones in my clothing. Through my clothes I have accompanied them to important events and have been a part of the memories one never forgets. I've experienced a connection that I have found particularly inspiring: I know these women understood my inherent desire for them to feel good about themselves and to tap into the power they have within them, which they control when they are confident. I learned early on that when I felt especially good as a result of how I had styled my own look head-to-toe, I owned the day. Many of the women I've met feel comfortable and familiar with me, as if I were a longtime friend. They know that I've thought about the things that are important to making them feel good, because they understand that I feel the same way, myself.

As a fashion designer, clothing has been my medium; however, beneath the clothing is a body and a spirit and a soul. Nearly forty years ago, I embarked upon

THIS IS MY PURPOSE.
HOW DO YOU FIND YOURS? IS IT INTUITIVE? IS IT THERE ALL ALONG? DOES IT REVEAL ITSELF? IS IT BIGGER THAN A DREAM?

a search to learn more about health and well-being, a journey that has reshaped how I lead my life. Since the opening of the Wellness Café in 2001, I have been sharing my insight and findings with everyone I can in order to bring the power of proactive well-being into the equation.

I have learned about the positive impact of a healthy lifestyle on aging, and this is where I am today. My purpose continues to evolve, and this book is part of it.

I not only want to wrap my arms around each of you through my clothing, but now I want to be sure that everything I know and everything I learn I share with you so you will own the power of a healthy body and mind. Then you can share it with your family and others you love and we can find a common ground of kindness and love for each other through the power of feeling good inside and out.

This is my purpose. How do you find yours? Is it intuitive? Is it there all along? Does it reveal itself? Is it bigger than a dream? And how do you know once you have found it? Well, it is partly intuitive and partly about answering this question: What do you do that can change the lives of those around you or the world you live in or, in fact, the world?

What impact do you want to have? What will make you fulfilled, energized, and inspired every day?

Living your purpose will make it possible to do all the things you need to do to reach the goals you need to reach in order to fulfill your dreams, which are as big as the world and as optimistic as your mind can imagine.   **NK**

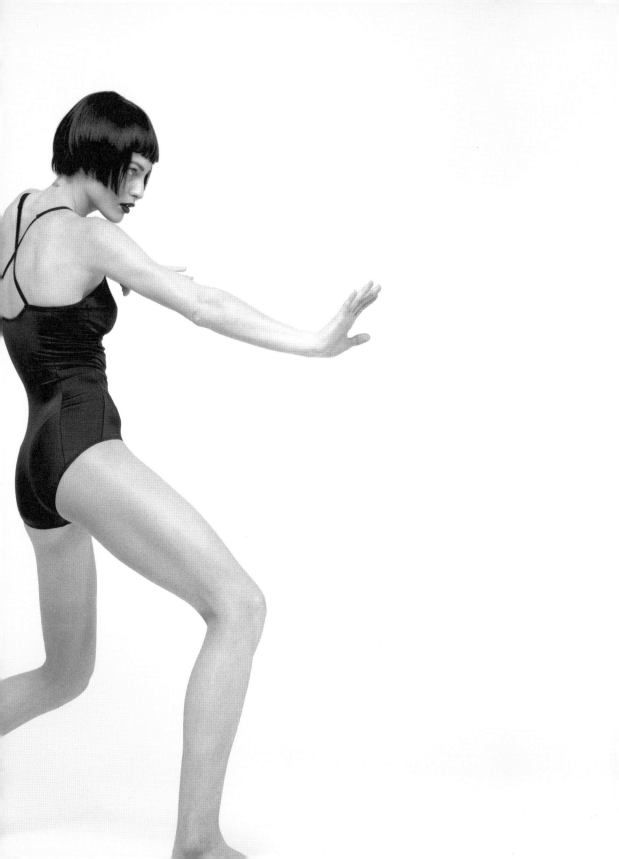

TEENs

Graduate from the Fashion Institute of Technology with a degree in Fashion Illustration.

Marry Mohammed Houssein Kamali.

First job: reservations agent at Northwest Orient Airlines, operating a Univac computer.

Start going to London—every weekend for four years.

20s

1967

The first KAMALI store opens at 229 East Fifty-Third Street, selling clothing brought from London.

1968

I start designing my own pieces: looks with elaborate appliqués, tie-die velvets, rhinestone-studded T-shirts, and hot pants—the first in NYC.

1973

The desire to design the vintage of the future leads me to create the All In One Dress and other multi-style jersey designs.

1974

Move shop to a second-floor space at 787 Madison Avenue.

The Parachute collection, made from actual silk parachutes. Diana Vreeland includes them in her Metropolitan Museum of Art Costume Institute curation looking at the future of fashion contrasted.

The Sleeping Bag Coat is born when I cut up my own sleeping bag after a camping trip.

30s

1975

Divorced.

1976

Farrah Fawcett wears her own red NK one-piece for her iconic swimsuit poster, photographed by Bruce McBroom and later considered the best-selling poster of all time.

Studio 54. Ian Schrager asks me to design the costume for Grace Jones's New Year's Eve performance, beginning a long friendship.

1977

On my own. OMO NORMA KAMALI opens at 6 West Fifty-Sixth Street.

My career as a swimwear designer is launched overnight by Francesco Scavullo's *Cosmo* cover of Christie Brinkley in the Pull Bikini.

1978

Costumes for the "Emerald City" sequence in Sidney Lumet's film *The Wiz*.

1980

Sweats: a new idea for active-casual fashion for day and night. Jones Apparel produces it. Lines at department stores form around the block.

1981

COTY Award for design innovation, celebrating the Sweats collection.

1982

A new license agreement begins in Japan and Hong Kong for the Sweats collection. It will last twenty-five years.

COTY Award for Women's Fashion Design.

Design and patent the high-heeled sneaker.

1983

I buy and redesign my own building at 11 West Fifty-Sixth Street. It will be my headquarters, retail store, design studio, and showroom going forward.

Earnie Award for Outstanding Children's Sportswear Design, celebrating the mini version of Sweats.

COTY Hall of Fame Award.

1984

"Fall Fantasy" video, which I write and produce, pioneers an important new direction in fashion marketing by embedding fashion into a story.

My research into the immune system, following the loss of friends to AIDS, begins a commitment to the importance of a healthy lifestyle.

40s

1985

Launch unisex fragrance collection: incense and perfume applied separately or layered for a customized scent.

My fashion films earn a Council of Fashion Designers of America Award.

Interiors magazine award for Best Retail Design.

Produce and direct "Fashion Aid" video for the Live Aid foundation to help fight famine in Africa.

1986

Honored by the Fashion Group's "salute to women who have made a difference in the fashion industry."

Costumes for choreographer Twyla Tharp's provocative and revolutionary dance *In The Upper Room* after an introduction from Richard Avedon. Twyla becomes a lifelong friend.

I create the Fashion Video Catalogue, a new merchandising tool that shows clothing in motion.

1987

Licensing agreement with Bloomingdale's for an exclusive collection. My "Sweet Dreams" video accompanies the launch.

Distinguished Architecture Award from the American Institute of Architects for the headquarters.

1988

OMO Home opens in SoHo.

Write and direct "The Reading of the Will," which wins an Award of Merit from the Video Culture International Video Competition.

1989

President George H. W. Bush presents me with the American Success Award for Vocational Technical Education at a White House ceremony in the Rose Garden.

1993

OMOgym activewear collection debuts at the first fashion shows at the Bryant Park tents. I feature thirty-five athletes from different sports as my runway models.

My entrée into beauty: the NORMA KAMALI skincare line, made with sea algae, enhances skin to replace makeup. I officially go foundation-free.

50s

1995

Launch modern lifestyle travel collection: twenty-five wash-and-wear, easy care, wrinkle-free styles, rolled into a reusable sack.

1996

www.normakamali.com launches with the presentation of my Fall 1996 collection: a virtual reality experience simultaneously broadcast for the Internet.

High school alumni Hall of Fame.

1998

Proud to be one of the first designers to launch e-commerce: 18008KAMALI becomes available for purchase online. "Shop Like a Celebrity" try-before-you-buy home service extended to all clients.

1999

Pencil Award for extraordinary commitment to New York City public school education.

2001

The events of 9/11 inspire me to open the Wellness Café.

Olive You line debuts after my olive orchard expedition through Europe.

The high-heeled sneaker is featured in the Met Costume Institute's "Extreme Beauty" exhibition.

2002

Fashion Group International's Entrepreneur Award.

Plaque on NYC's Fashion Walk of Fame.

2004

Transform the headquarters, painting it white inside and out.

www.barxv.com launches, offering the full line of products from the Wellness Café.

Wellness nights at the Wellness Café: restorative yoga, tai chi, Pilates, and Gyrokinesis, with teas, talks, and tastings.

60s

2005

CFDA Board of Directors Special Tribute Award.

2008

Ink deal with Walmart to design a collection of classics, all priced under $20.

2009

Launch of the Norma Kamali iPhone app at the SoHo Apple store with accompanying presentation "The Democratization of Fashion and How Technology Is Changing Fashion Presentations." We provide customers access through QR codes and direct video interaction.

Fashion Designer of the Year at the American Apparel and Footwear Association's American Image Awards.

2010

ScanLife barcodes allow shoppers to buy direct off of mannequins and through our store windows.

Named to CFDA Board of Directors.

Commencement speaker at FIT's Fiftieth Anniversary, where I receive an honorary doctorate.

Begin microsite e-blasts, which became a preferred direct-to-consumer sales method.

"Conversation with Norma Kamali," part of the Museum of Modern Art's wellness conference.

2011

Farrah Fawcett's original red swimsuit is donated to the Smithsonian Institute.

2012

Stop Objectification Campaign begins.

"Hey Baby" radio special on Sirius XM brings awareness to the objectification of women.

Kamalikulture—all styles under $100—launches on Amazon and Zappos.

Team up with the American Federation of Teachers at their Detroit Convention to present a fashion show featuring affordable fashion for teachers, with members as models.

2013

Tribeca Disruptive Innovation Award.

JP Morgan empowerment talk discussing workplace objectification streamed globally.

Hey Baby film, promoting the Stop Objectification Campaign, is presented at the American Public Health Film Festival.

2014

Re:gender Forbes Summit with a Fire Starter Award for advocacy of women's empowerment.

Design carpets for "Weaving for a Brighter Future," handmade by Taliban widows who receive health care and education for their children.

Exclusive distribution through e-commerce continues to expand across Europe, Asia, and the Middle East.

70s

2015

The Sleeping Bag Coat is included in the Met Costume Institute's "Jacqueline de Ribes: The Art of Style" exhibition.

CFDA Geoffrey Beene Lifetime Achievement Award.

2016

Publication of *Facing East*, an accupunture handbook written with Dr. Jingduan Yang.

National Arts Club Medal of Honor for fashion design.

Seriously?, my ongoing Sirius XM series on women, begins.

Exhibition at the Tampa Museum of Art celebrating my career.

2017

NORMALIFE! podcast launches. Guests share stories, expertise, and motivation for a healthy lifestyle.

The Museum of Modern Art includes the Sleeping Bag Coat in "Items: Is Fashion Modern?" an exhibition, featuring 111 styles that still hold currency.

2018

Both men and women model my Spring 2019 collection, marking our official move to gender fluidity. Clothes no longer define the person; the person defines the style.

2019

Launch of NORMALIFE, as a democratic and inclusive line of personal care products based upon the three pillars of a healthy lifestyle.

2020

Covid-19 leads me to rethink the future of fashion, and my company, yet again, Reinvention, here I come.

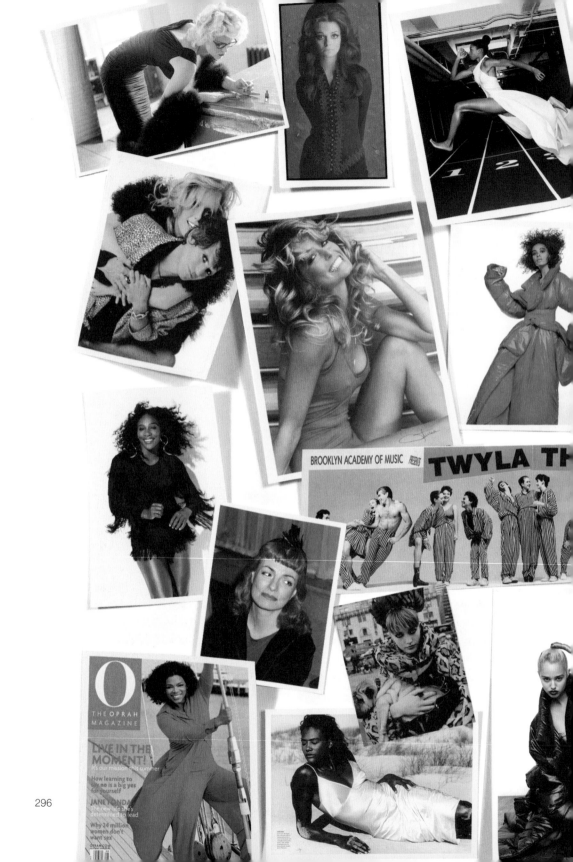

BROOKLYN ACADEMY OF MUSIC PRESENTS TWYLA TH

296

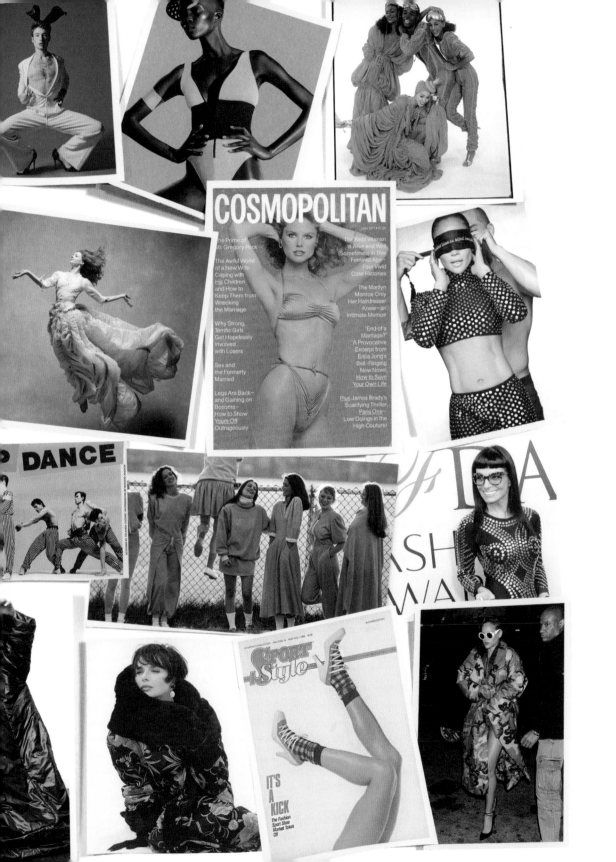

COSMOPOLITAN

The Prime of
Mr. Gregory Peck

The Awful World
of a New Wife
Coping with
His Children
and How to
Keep Them from
Wrecking
the Marriage

Why Strong,
Terrific Girls
Get Hopelessly
Involved
with Losers

Sex and
the Formerly
Married

Legs Are Back—
and Gaining on
Bosoms—
How to Show
Yours Off
Outrageously

The Real Woman
Is Alive and Well
(Sometimes) in This
Feminist Age—
Four Vivid
Case Histories

The Marilyn
Monroe Only
Her Hairdresser
Knew—an
Intimate Memoir

"End of a
Marriage?"
A Provocative
Excerpt from
Erica Jong's
Bell-Ringing
New Novel,
How to Save
Your Own Life

Plus James Brady's
Scarifying Thriller,
Paris One—
Low Doings in the
High Couture!

DANCE

FASH WA

Sport Style

IT'S A KICK
The Fashion
Sport Shoe
Market Takes
Off

RESOURCES

EXPERTS & ORGANIZATIONS TO KNOW

Andrew Weil, MD,
integrative health expert;
www.drweil.com

Tieraona Low Dog, MD,
integrative health and **herbal medicine
expert**; *www.drlowgod.com*

Drew Ramsey, MD,
psychiatrist, farmer, and founder of the
Brain Food Health Clinic, New York;
www.drewramseymd.com

Jingduan Yang, MD, FAPA,
**acupuncture and Chinese medicine
expert**, integrative mental health
specialist and psychiatrist,
Yang Institute of Integrative Medicine;
www.yanginstitute.com

Abdi Assadi,
acupuncturist, **spiritual counselor
and healer**; *www.abdiassadi.com*

Nir Barzilai, MD,
longevity expert and director of the
Institute for Aging Research at the
Albert Einstein College of Medicine;
www.einstein.yu.edu

Orli Etigin, MD,
internal medicine and women's health,
Weill Cornell Medicine;
www.weillcornell.org/oretingin

Rebecca Brightman, MD,
obstetrics, gynecology, **reproductive
science and menopause**, Mount Sinai;
*www.mountsinai.org/profiles/
rebecca-c-brightman*

Dena Harris, MD,
gynecologist and **bioidentical
hormone replacement therapy**
specialist, Maiden Lane Medical, NYC;
*www.maidenlanemedical.com/profile/
dena-harris-md/*

The **North American Menopause
Society**, for information on mental
well-being and physical health.
www.menopause.org

MGH Center for Women's Mental
Health: **reproductive psychiatry** and
support for women's emotional
well-being across their life cycle.
www.womensmentalhealth.org

Julia Smith, MD, PhD,
medical oncology, **breast cancer
specialist**, NYU Langone Perlmutter
Cancer Center;
*www.nyulangone.org/
doctors/1114963907/julia-a-smith*

Amy Tiersten, MD,
hematology and medical oncology;
breast cancer specialist,
Dubin Breast Center, Mount Sinai;
*www.mountsinai.org/profiles/
amy-tiersten*

Joseph Lane, MD,
orthopedic surgeon, specialist
in **metabolic bone health** and
osteoporosis, Hospital for Special
Surgery and New York Presbyterian;
*www.hss.edu/physicians_
lane-joseph.asp*

National Osteoporosis Foundation,
for information women of every
age should know, and for help locating
a professional.
www.nof.org

Sleep health information,
guidelines and lifestyle ideas from
the National Sleep Foundation:
www.sleep.org and
www.sleepfoundation.org

Ellen Gendler, MD,
medical and cosmetic **dermatology**;
www.genderdermatology.com

Gregg Litchuy, DDS,
medical and cosmetic **dentistry**;
www.lowenberglituchykantor.com

Gilles Baudin,
Thai yoga massage;
www.hamptons-thai-yogamassage.com

Barbara Reeder,
spiritual medium available for
in-person appointments and tele-
consultations;
Angelic_Intuitive@aol.com

Karen Thorne,
astrologer and psychic available
for in-person appointments and
tele-consultations;
www.karenthrone.com

Clean beauty reference: Environmental
Working Group's Skin Deep ingredient
and product guide:
www.ewg.org/skindeep/

Information on **GMOs and food**:
Non-GMO Project;
www.nongmoproject.org

What's in Your Food? Environmental
Working Group's **GMO Guide**;
*www.ewg.org/research/
shoppers-guide-to-avoiding-gmos*

**National Eating Disorders
Association** (NEDA);
www.nationaleatingdisorders.org;
Helpline: *(800) 223-7931*

The Me Too Movement's **Advocacy
Resource Library**, for support, legal
resources, and help reporting
and handling **objectification**, **sexual
violence and assault**.
*www.metoomvmt.org/advocacy-
resources-library/national-resources/*

**U.S Equal Employment Opportunity
Commission**, resource for employment
discrimination; *www.eeoc.gov*

RESOURCES

NK BOOK CLUB

Facing East: Ancient Health and Beauty Secrets for the Modern Age, Jingduan Yang, MD, FAPA, and Norma Kamali

Healthy Aging: A Lifelong Guide to Your Well-Being, Andrew Weil, MD

Natural Health, Natural Medicine: The Complete Guide to Wellness and Self-Care for Optimum Health, Andrew Weil, MD

Life Is Your Best Medicine: A Woman's Guide to Health, Healing, and Wholeness at Every Age, Tieraona Low Dog, MD

Rejuvenation: A Wellness Guide for Women and Men, Horst Rechelbacher

Herbal Antibiotics: Natural Alternatives for Treating Drug-Resistant Bacteria, Stephen Harrod Buhner

Shadows on the Path, Abdi Assadi

Healthy Gut, Flat Stomach: The Fast and Easy Low-FODMAP Diet Plan, Danielle Capalino, MSPH, RD

In Defense of Food: An Eater's Manifesto, Michael Pollan

The Complete Guide to Fasting: Heal Your Body Through Intermittent, Alternate-Day, and Extended Fasting, Jason Fung, MD, with Jimmy Moore

One Simple Thing: A New Look at the Science of Yoga and How it Can Transform Your Life, Eddie Stern

Science of Yoga: Understand the Anatomy and Physiology to Perfect Your Practice, Ann Swanson

RECOMMENDED FILMS

Practicing Mindfulness: An Introduction to Meditation

Supercharge Your Immune System

In Defense of Food

Forks Over Knives

Food, Inc.

What the Health

The Truth About Alcohol

I WAS LUCKY TO BE DRAWN BY THE LEGENDARY FASHION ILLUSTRATOR ANTONIO LOPEZ.

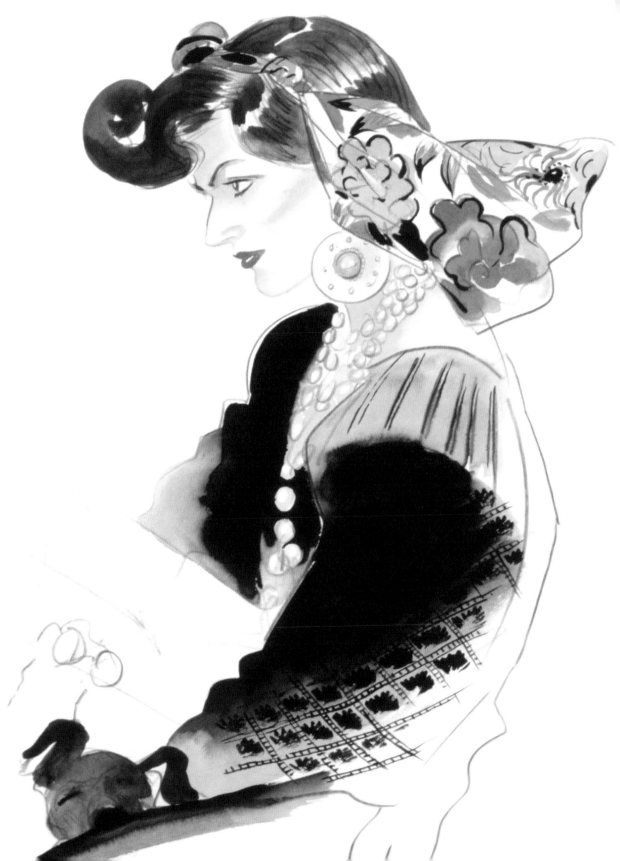

I OWE MANY THANKS TO ALL THE FOLKS THROUGHOUT MY CAREER WHO BELIEVED IN MY WORK AND INSPIRED ME TO KEEP LIVING MY DREAM.

THANK YOU TO

ELVIS, for buying multiples of the same white gowns through the years for the women in his life.

RAQUEL WELCH, for inviting me to design red carpet looks for her, year after year, on a body that was cultivated to perfection.

VOGUE and ***HARPER'S BAZAAR***, for recognizing my talent six months from my first day as a designer in business, giving me full-page editorials.

JACKIE BISSET, for looking amazing in **PETER GUBER**'s film *The Deep*, in my white T-shirt swimsuit (which inspired wet T-shirt contests for years), and thanks to **PETER** and **TARA** for being super-supporters.

SLY STONE, for buying multiple brightly colored feather jackets for his performances.

CHER, for being one of the most beautiful, untraditional beauties of our time and for buying so many clothes, and in turn helping me pay the rent.

ROBERT DE NIRO, for shopping for my favorite model in the 1980s, **TOUKIE SMITH**.

DIANA ROSS, for rocking gowns I made for her with as much drama as I could imagine, trying to match her dynamic performances.

JOEL SCHUMACHER and **SIDNEY LUMET**, for inviting me to design costumes for the "Emerald City" sequence in *The Wiz*.

JOHN LENNON, for shopping with **YOKO** and being soooo charming, funny, and brilliant.

BETTE MIDLER, the super-talented, generous, funny human, for finding me early on in our careers and inviting me to help her design some of the powerful Bette looks in their raw early stages. And in memory of **JEANINE**.

THE NEW YORK DOLLS, for finding my clothes and styling themselves into the New York scene.

DR. ANDREW WEIL, for opening up the world of healthy lifestyle to me almost thirty years ago.

KAMA PERSAUD, who has been with me for forty-seven years, who has sewn every significant new design, and whom I love very much.

SCAVULLO, for launching me into the swimwear business with a *Cosmo* swim cover of newcomer **CHRISTIE BRINKLEY**, thx to **SEAN BYRNES**.

ROD STEWART, for tirelessly shopping for frocks and shooooes for the women in his life.

MADONNA, for some of my favorite photos of any celeb in my clothing through the years, especially the pieces I designed for *Vanity Fair*, shot by **STEVEN MEISEL**.

DIANA VREELAND, for inviting me to create parachutes for the first Metropolitan Museum of Art Costume Institute exhibition including designers of the current time.

RICHARD AVEDON, for introducing me to **TWYLA THARP**, who offered me the honor of collaborating with her on nine dances to date, especially one of my favorites, *In the Upper Room*.

IAN SCHRAGER, for inviting me to design costumes for the first big New Year's Eve party at Studio 54, for the **GRACE JONES** performance … Then becoming my best friend and biggest supporter. And for introducing me to my soul mate, **MARTY EDELMAN**.

HORST RECHELBACHER, the founder of Aveda, who influenced and reinforced my commitment to safety and beauty for women.

JOAN JETT, for letting me have so much fun with leather and her Elvis looks.

WHITNEY HOUSTON, for the ease and elegance with which she wore my swimwear and clothing.

VINNY PASCAL, a friend since we were sixteen, for posing for me while I sketched him to exhaustion.

FARRAH FAWCETT, for having my red swimsuit in her bag when she shot her famous poster.

VICTOR HUGO, Halston's collaborator, for knocking off my swimsuit (his version of which appeared on the cover of *Time* magazine), and then paying me back by introducing me to parachutes!!

EDDIE KAMALI, for selling clothes for ten times the price I thought anyone should pay for my first designs.

DIANE EDWARDS, for sharing a fun history with me in London through the sixties, one of the most powerfully exciting times in my life.

DR. JINGDUAN YANG, my teacher and friend, who continues to teach me the benefits of Eastern Medicine and acupuncture.

MARY LOU LUTHER and **ARTHUR**, for helping to get me sewing machines when I decided to go out on my own.

SIDNEY KIMMEL, who, with blind faith in my sweats, signed a deal with me and never saw a sample.

BOB CURRIE, for camping with me and being part of the discovery of the Sleeping Bag Coat.

ELIZABETH RACINE, my mentor and sister in life.

LADY GAGA, for wearing the wedding gown I designed for her mother in 1983 in a music video.

BEYONCÉ, for wearing my clothes since Destiny's Child and looking more and more beautiful.

ETTA JAMES, for her inspiration and friendship, making anything for her for the pure joy and worship of her talent.

RIHANNA, for looking amazing in everyone's clothing, and even some of mine, from my Sleeping Bag Coat to fringe.

JENNIFER LOPEZ, for looking fantastic in my favorite swim photos ever.

MICHELLE OBAMA, for wearing multiple NK travel sets on her book tour.

JENNIFER WALSH, for encouraging me to tell my story.

The team at **WME**.

REBECCA KAPLAN at Abrams.

EMILY WARDWELL, for a beautifully designed book.

SARAH BROWN, for making sure my voice and message were clear and authentic in this book.

Parts of the above are adapted from Norma's acceptance speech upon receiving her Lifetime Achievement Award from the CFDA in 2016.

Editor: Rebecca Kaplan
Designer: Emily Wardwell
Production Manager: Anet Sirna-Bruder

Library of Congress Control Number: 2020931057

ISBN: 978-1-4197-4740-3
eISBN: 978-1-64700-019-6

Printed and bound in the United States
10 9 8 7 6 5 4 3

Every reasonable attempt has been made to obtain copyright information and permissions for all images used herein. If there are any omissions, Abrams will be happy to add appropriate acknowledgment to future printings.

Abrams books are available at special discounts when purchased in quantity for premiums and promotions as well as fundraising or educational use. Special editions can also be created to specification. For details, contact specialsales@abramsbooks.com or the address below.

Abrams® is a registered trademark of Harry N. Abrams, Inc.

ABRAMS The Art of Books
195 Broadway, New York, NY 10007
abramsbooks.com